THE
FLEXIBLE
BODY

First published in the United Kingdom in 2018 by
Pavilion
43 Great Ormond Street
London
WC1N 3HZ

ISBN 978-1-91121-694-0

A CIP catalogue record for this book is available from the British Library.

10 9 8 7 6 5 4 3 2

Reproduction by Rival Colour Ltd, UK
Printed and bound by GPS Group, Slovenia

This book can be ordered direct from the publisher at
www.pavilionbooks.com

Note
The information in this book is not intended as a substitute for professional
medical advice and treatment. If you have an existing injury or any medical
conditions, it is recommended that you consult a medical professional
before following any of the information or exercises contained in this book.
Care should be taken at all times when using furniture and fittings around
the home to achieve a movement. Always check that items used for support
are stable. Neither the author nor the publisher can accept responsibility
for any injury or illness that may arise as a result of following the advice
contained in this work. Any application of the information contained in this
book is at the reader's sole discretion.

Photography by Tom Leighton

THE FLEXIBLE BODY

MOVE BETTER ANYWHERE ANYTIME IN 10 MINUTES A DAY

ROGER FRAMPTON

PAVILION

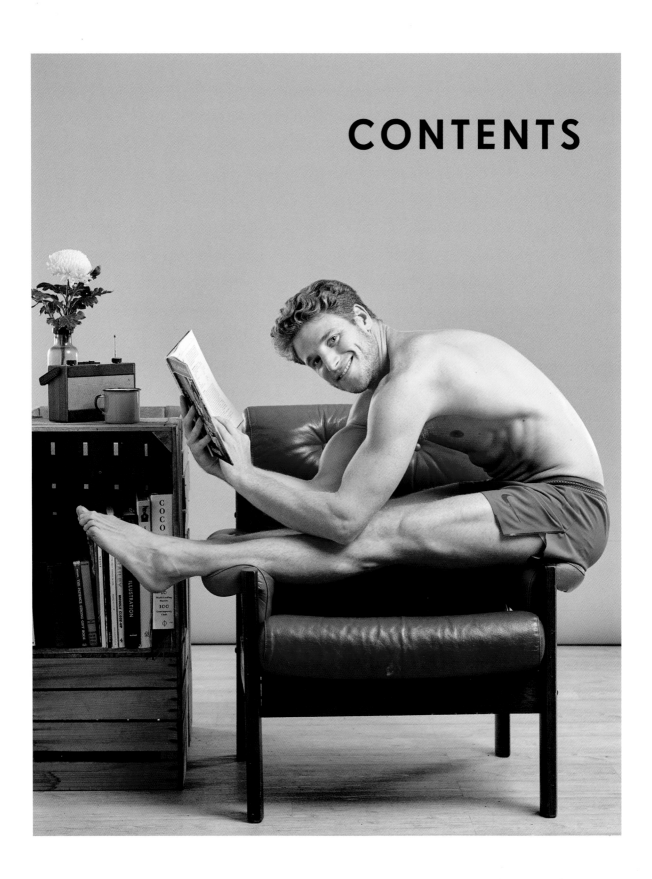

CONTENTS

How to Use this Book   6

Your Movement Plan   8

THE METHOD

The Frampton Method   12

Debunking Exercise   14

Movement First   20

A, B, C, D, E of Longevity   22

The Frampton Phrasebook   28

THE MOVES

Overhead Squat   32

Front Support   44

Hollow Body   56

Frog Stand   70

Legs, Legs, Legs   84

Hip Action   98

Headstand   112

L-Sits   128

Stair Bridge   140

Index   154

My Story   156

Thank you!   160

HOW TO USE THIS BOOK

You can achieve every exercise in this book at home and without the need for equipment. I suggest using mats, carpets, rugs, blocks, books and chairs in some exercises to make them a little easier but there's nothing to stop you starting right now! It's all about your body.

Half the exercises in the book are static and half are slow and controlled movements that help you to develop strength and flexibility in the right places. Working at this pace gives you time to focus on being fully conscious, as well as allowing you to find flaws and weaknesses in your movement.

The book contains nine "moves" that you have a lifetime to master. However you need to complete 10 minutes a day. Every day! Each move is made up of ten support exercises, arranged by level of difficulty, 1 being the easiest and 10 the hardest. and each support exercise is subdivided into a 1-minute controlled movement and a 1-minute static hold.

CHECK YOURSELF BEFORE YOU WRECK YOURSELF

Freeze! Right now! Don't move a muscle. Now, check yourself. What is your body doing in this current position? How are you holding your foot, neck, hands, feet? Are you leaning to one side, forward or back; left or right? Don't judge or try to change it, just notice it. This is your default position in this moment in time. Get used to identifying all these postural habits because it will give you a good idea of what to look out for when training. REMEMBER: stay conscious of your body as much as you can. The more aware you become of your body outside of training, the more aware you'll become during training, too.

BEFORE YOU START

The first thing you need to do is to find what level you're at with all nine moves. Start at exercise 1 and see how many support exercises you can complete within each move before the movement or hold becomes unachievable.

The support exercise before the one that becomes unachievable is your current level of ability and you should practise this exercise until you can achieve it for the required time before moving onto the next support exercise. By the time you complete the support exercises, you will be able to tackle the move shown at the beginning of each chapter.

Keep track of your ability as you work through the exercises. For example, in the Overhead Squat, if I can get my heels to the floor but I can't yet stay there for the full minute then I will work on support exercise 4. The Overhead Squat is move 1. The support exercise is number 4. Write it down like this... **1/4**.

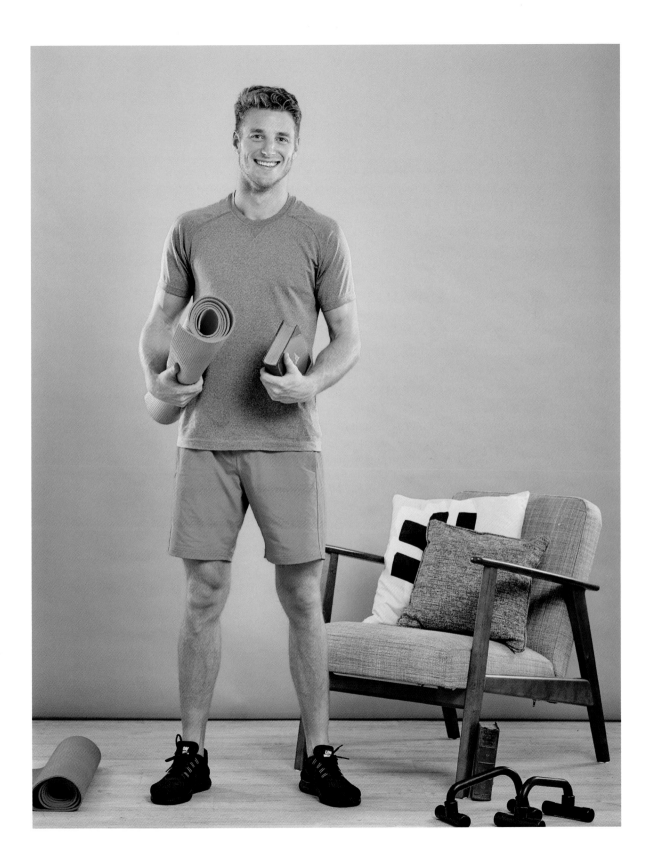

YOUR MOVEMENT PLAN

You've picked up this book – CONGRATULATIONS! This is a movement plan for life. By following the exercises in this book for just 10 minutes a day you will keep your body healthy and mobile.

DAILY TRAINING

Aim to complete 10 minutes of exercise altogether. That's all – 10 minutes. To make up those 10 minutes, choose five exercises from the book and perform a 1-minute movement and a 1-minute hold for each. Choose support exercises that you are able to complete. If you can't complete either the movement or the static hold, you need to step back to an earlier support exercise that is manageable for you. Don't rush. Slowly, your movement will improve so that you can then challenge yourself to progress to the next step. Don't skip steps or kid yourself you're there when you're not. If you have mastered an exercise, you'll be able to hold the exact position for 1 minute without moving. Only at that point are you ready to move on.

BUILD YOUR WEEK

Using the chart opposite, build your own personalised week of training. If you followed the instructions on page 6, you should now have nine exercises written down that you need to work on, each containing a 1-minute movement and a 1-minute hold that looks something like this; **1/4, 2/3, 3/5, 4/2, 5/4, 6/4, 7/1, 8/3, 9/1**. Now write these into your chart on the right day.

REMEMBER: the second number is personal to you depending on what support exercise you are on. Write down your first move/level on the day you are going to start.

For example, if I'm starting on Tuesday my five entries will be: **1/4, 2/3, 3/5, 4/2, 5/4**. This will be your 10-minute training for Tuesday. Your Wednesday will continue like so: **6/4, 7/1, 8/3, 9/1, 1/4**. (See how you continued back to move 1 again.) Keep repeating this until your chart is completely full! This will set you up for your training for the next 7 days.

As you work through your movement journey, you will find you progress and your ability improves so after a few days, weeks or months **1/4** becomes **1/5** and you'll need to edit your chart as this happens.

Don't read any further until you have your plan for the next seven days in place. Remember you're only committing to 10 minutes a day. (That's around three advert breaks.)

Let's get moving!

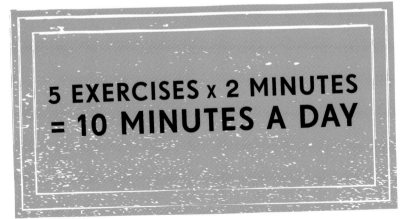

5 EXERCISES x 2 MINUTES = 10 MINUTES A DAY

	1.	**2.**	**3.**	**4.**	**5.**
Monday	Move / Level _____/_____	Move / Level _____/_____	Move / Level _____/_____	Move / Level _____/_____	Move / Level _____/_____
Tuesday	Move / Level _____/_____	Move / Level _____/_____	Move / Level _____/_____	Move / Level _____/_____	Move / Level _____/_____
Wednesday	Move / Level _____/_____	Move / Level _____/_____	Move / Level _____/_____	Move / Level _____/_____	Move / Level _____/_____
Thursday	Move / Level _____/_____	Move / Level _____/_____	Move / Level _____/_____	Move / Level _____/_____	Move / Level _____/_____
Friday	Move / Level _____/_____	Move / Level _____/_____	Move / Level _____/_____	Move / Level _____/_____	Move / Level _____/_____
Saturday	Move / Level _____/_____	Move / Level _____/_____	Move / Level _____/_____	Move / Level _____/_____	Move / Level _____/_____
Sunday	Move / Level _____/_____	Move / Level _____/_____	Move / Level _____/_____	Move / Level _____/_____	Move / Level _____/_____

(You might want to photocopy this page before you write in your chart. If you need a spare copy there is a free PDF at www.roger.coach.)

QUESTIONS TO ASK YOURSELF

Did I feel anything in my body?
Can I name the movement as either "good feeling" or "pain"?
What level of intensity was the feeling or pain?
Was the exercise challenging enough?

THE

METHOD

THE FRAMPTON METHOD

In these next pages, I am going to explain why exercise is not what you think it is. I'll explain why conscious, slow, deliberate movement is the way to get your body back. But first, what is the Frampton Method?

» I believe that as kids we all taught ourselves to move perfectly.

» I believe the key to wellness is relearning how our bodies were designed to move.

» I believe the pain we feel in our bodies will dissipate as a result of moving like we once could.

» I believe we should all be able to access the hidden potential our bodies hold...

I also believe that the best results take time. The Frampton Method is not a quick fix. It is a programme of training for long-term benefit. Imagine being in a maths class as a kid and the teacher setting a test, then screaming "Go! Go! Go!" You might complete the paper, but have you sacrificed the quality of your work and used your full capacity? Or, do you have a sense of relief that it's over? The skills that teach you how to hold yourself in a Headstand are techniques worth learning properly and then applying consciously. They are the foundations of how your body moves and works at its best. If you take the time to learn and apply them, you get the best results.

USE IT, OR LOSE IT

Think of the stiffness you see in the older generation as they walk around you – do you think that was how they were born?

Think of your own range of movement compared with how you could move as a child, or even a mere 10 years ago.

The fitness industry's answer to our stiffness is to get us out and about and moving... I agree. However, we do not need to move *more*! If we simply move more, we'll just repeat the same movement patterns over and over again that led to our restricted movement in the first place.

Rather than moving more, each of us needs to move as our bodies were designed to move. We need to reverse engineer the process to reinstate the full range of movement before it disappears forever.

Move better and more regularly and you will:
» Burn fat
» Improve health
» Feel confident
» Avoid injury
» Lose weight
» Live longer

The Frampton Method is a "movement first" philosophy. Exercise is a "learning" process, measuring progress through your understanding of how your body moves best and applying that understanding appropriately. My aim is to teach you how to hold specific body positions and to be able to move as you once could.

Think of it like this:

If your house were burgled, you could try to find the perpetrator, knocking on doors, but leaving your house as susceptible to burglary as it was before. Or, you accept that it's happened and set about tightening up security so that it doesn't happen again.

Now apply this analogy to your body. You have an injury or pain. You can either knock on the door of every doctor or specialist and try to find a quick fix, or you can accept that it's happened and set about making your body the most resilient it can be so that you can move without pain again.

The catalyst for your pain is a poor pattern of movement.

The Frampton Method teaches you patterns of movement that have long-term benefits for your body. It is a masterclass in the essential movements we were born with, combining elements of gymnastic fundamentals with using the full consciousness of the mind.

I strongly believe that you will need nothing other than your own body (and patience, awareness and – okay – perhaps a few household props) to transform your ability to move. It's time to stop looking for excuses and unveil the true power of your phenomenal machine: the human body.

PAIN PROTECTS YOUR SPINE!

The most important training tool in your learning is your spine. Consider the possibility that the body is essentially just the spine and each segment of the spine is designed to move in a particular way.

If a segment of the spine were to "lose" its ability to move in the way it was designed to move, something further down the chain must be affected. The spine cannot lose function; it is the body's utmost priority, to be protected at all costs.

So, when you feel tight hamstrings, lower back pain or neck pain, the feelings and symptoms are all just clever compensation mechanisms that your body is using to protect the spine to keep you functioning.

In other words, your body will happily pay the cost of a shoulder or hip injury in order to protect your central movement mechanism: the spine. Any pain you feel anywhere in the body is there to keep you moving and keep you alive.

DEBUNKING EXERCISE

Okay, let's look at the three main reasons I hear for why people exercise – and why, to my mind, they leave you chasing the mythical pot of gold at the end of the rainbow (that is, they are a waste of time as reasons go).

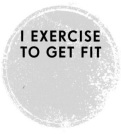

I EXERCISE TO GET FIT

It's not your fault if you give this answer. It's an industry-standard answer. When I first qualified as a personal trainer, I'd run all sorts of tests to see how fit people were. It seemed to make sense at the time: take a measure of ability, then repeat the test at a later date to see if the results of that measure have improved.

So why is this way of testing fitness flawed?

Human physiology is extremely complex; we are machines capable of *billions* and *billions* of movements. If a whole industry is using the same standard exercises as tests for how "fit" we are, then we're only seeing how "fit" people are at the tests that are being given. We're not *necessarily* improving. Just because we did an extra five jumps in that minute doesn't mean every jump was identical. For example, if burpee 1 didn't look identical to burpee 10, then perhaps we didn't do 10 burpees. This is a classic example of *how much* you move rather than *how* you move.

What if you run so much that you lose the ability to touch your toes? Surely you've just compensated for one weakness with another. According to the industry you're fitter than you were, but are you now at a higher risk of injury because you lack movement in a part of the body you haven't trained while running?

Do you believe that one day Mo Farah just started running faster and faster? Hell no. It's his job. He has a coach; he uses specific techniques; and he runs in a way that is efficient and can bring home gold medals. But is he generally fit? Would he come in the top three in an Olympic 100-metre sprint? If we put Mo on some gymnastic rings, how would he fare? We can't say he is simply "fit". We have to say that he is fit at what he does. So, when you say, "I want to get fit", I say "Get fit at what?"

I EXERCISE TO KEEP IN SHAPE

To keep in whose shape? If it's your shape, you're already "in shape". Unless, that is, you have some idea of the shape you should be in, in which case it's an ideal. So, at this point you'll want to show me some pictures of models or movie stars in the shape you're aiming for. I've worked alongside some of the most high-profile male and female models in the world, and if you think for one second these people are constantly happy with their bodies, you're mistaken. Trying to look like them when they don't necessarily even like their own body is a fast track to your own body misery. If you base your goals on an image, you'll never be happy. You'll always want more. What you see in the mirror will never be good enough.

And there's another thing – who says what's "in shape" anyway? Over time and across cultures, in shape is fashion- and trend-based, which means it's pretty fickle and ever-changing. Look at images of people in the 1970s – being so-called in shape then gave a completely different look to how it does now. Similarly, culturally in shape differs wildly. The Japanese have a certain physique they would call in shape, as do the Russians, and I assure you these are not the same. I'm sorry to disappoint you, but you can never train to be in shape, because being in shape is purely down to perception. For the purposes of this book, the only aspiration you should have is to go back to having the range of movement you had as a child – not anyone else as a child (or an adult), but you.

I EXERCISE TO LOSE WEIGHT

Unless you were born with a relevant medical condition, no one is born overweight. Ricky Gervais summed up the weight issue perfectly in his stand-up routine:

"YOU get fat if YOU take in more calories than YOU burn off."

This has absolutely nothing whatsoever to do with exercise quality. If *you* eat (input) more than *you* move (output), then *you* put on weight. But moving more doesn't necessarily equate to moving better. Think about this...

» If I banged my head on a brick wall, would I be burning calories? **Yes.**
» Would my fitness app congratulate me on banging my head against a brick wall and count it as output? **Yes.**
» Would my heart rate rise as a result of banging my head on a brick wall? **Yes.**
» Am I moving more? **Yes.**
» Would I lose weight? **Eventually, yes.**

So, in the eyes of the fitness industry everything adds up. But you and I both know that repeatedly banging my head against a brick wall isn't healthy. So what if I've lost weight? I now have a long-term head injury.

Never use exercise to "fix" a weight problem. If you're exercising with the sole purpose of losing weight, you're just sacrificing your ability to move better in order to be thinner. You're just swapping one problem for another. Why? Because you're focusing on losing weight and not on how you move.

FITNESS VS MOVEMENT

On the left are fitness statements, and on the right are the equivalents for movement. They show why movement is more sustainable in the long term.

I train muscles	My body was designed to move in a specific way. The more I keep in line with how I'm designed to move, the less I need to focus on building muscles and the more naturally lean I will become anyway.
I want to lose weight	The more complex movements I learn and apply, the quicker my body will start burning fat at a high rate. (More on this shortly.)
I want to burn more calories	As I work my way through the exercise progressions in the book, the number of calories I burn will increase.
I want to move as fast as I can	The slower I move, the more conscious I become of my body; the more conscious I am of my body, the quicker I will progress and the more self-aware I will become.
I want a better butt	If I take my time to learn specific movements, my butt will become more toned and powerful.
I do	I learn.
I want a better body	My body is perfect just the way it is. My body will change as I progress. (Again, more on that shortly.)

This book strips away old-school "fitness" terminology and gives a new, fresh approach. Learning is the new doing. Exercise stops being exercise as we know it, and instead teaches us new skills, new ways of *moving* and *focusing* that stay with us and benefit us for the rest of our lives. Think mindfulness meets exercise.

In short, the skills you'll learn in this book will not only teach your body new motor skills, but also enable you to develop phenomenal core strength, a greater understanding of how your body moves and greater powers of concentration.

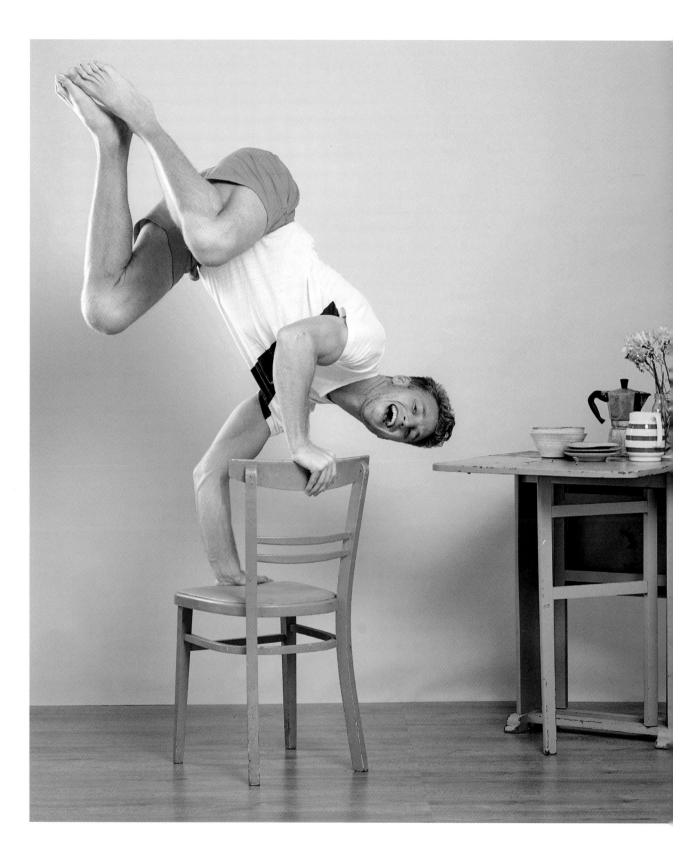

WHAT ABOUT NUTRITION?

I don't believe I have a diet. Well, not a diet in the sense of eating more to gain muscle or eating less to lose weight. I see diet another way.

I think diet should be something that is sustainable for life. I've eaten the same way for many years, even if I have a shoot coming up that I need to look good for. My body stays pretty much the same all year round. The only way it sometimes changes is if I add more flexibility or strength into my training. My physique is always a by-product of the exercise that I'm doing.

I've trained with some of the top gymnastic coaches in the world, and listened to some of the greatest acrobats, all of whom follow the same regime: they don't diet; they just have a strict training programme. For me, nutrition shouldn't even be put in the same category as exercise. It's like putting English and Science together. They're called different things for a reason.

Exercise is exercise and nutrition is nutrition. I've met nutritionists who have preached to me about what I should put in my body when they can't even sit in a squat. If abs were made in the kitchen, the top athletes in the world would spend their time at home, but they don't.

Why? Because:
» Eating broccoli won't help you to learn to do a Headstand.
» Eating quinoa won't improve your leg flexibility.
» Courgetti will not improve your wrist movement.

Are you following? Now, I'm not arguing that some foods aren't good for your body – I'm saying they have nothing to do with the way you move.

CONSCIOUS MOVEMENT

So, if all those reasons for exercising are a waste of time, what's the alternative? Answer: conscious movement and using the "movement first" philosophy (see page 20).

Let's first look at some everyday exercises that many of us do without really giving them a second thought – this is what I call *unconscious* exercise. Take squats, planks and press-ups. The short-term effects of pumping these out in endless repetition might look good, but in the long run, are those unconscious reps really doing you any good? Here's what I think:

» Squats can give you great legs, but are they just creating tightness and restriction in your hips from repeated one-directional movement?

» Planks can give you great abs, but what are they doing to the muscles in your stomach and lower back that you might be ignoring?
» Press-ups can give you a great chest and arms, but are they restricting movement in your shoulders?

Thing is, I'm not interested in short-term gain. I think unconscious exercise (in not focussing on how you move) is a form of self-harm. Yes, self-harm. If you're doing something to yourself that gives you short-term reward but causes you long-term damage, then you are self-harming.

Let me explain this another way. If you spend the majority of your day in static positions, but have a body that's designed for constant movement, then you're living outside of your means. You are in debt to your body and owe it a life of movement.

The answer is to forget quick-fix, short-term strategies and instead learn movements that do good in the long term. This means focusing on and being fully conscious of the specific movements you are doing. This is the founding principle of the Frampton Method. Everything you do in this book, you need to do with pure consciousness. By doing this, you will achieve a strong, restriction-free body without causing yourself long-term damage.

There are no quick fixes, but in time you will:
» Get fit (give your body back its movement)
» Lose weight (burn fat)
» Get in shape (*your* shape)

Sound familiar? I never train to change the appearance of my body. I'm not trying to gain muscle or lose weight or aspire to be like anyone else. All I'm trying to do is get back the beautiful essence of movement I was born with. I use Handstand techniques I've learned from gymnastics, some stretches from yoga classes, some moves I've created myself. I'm neither a yogi nor a gymnast. I refuse to be confined within any discipline. I am a human

and the Frampton Method is, quite simply, human movement. I'm going to teach you how to move your body. As by-products I promise you this: becoming fit will occur, changing shape will occur and weight loss will occur – but none of these is ever the goal. They all happen as a result of conscious movement.

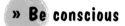

» Be conscious

» Move consciously

» Live phenomenally!

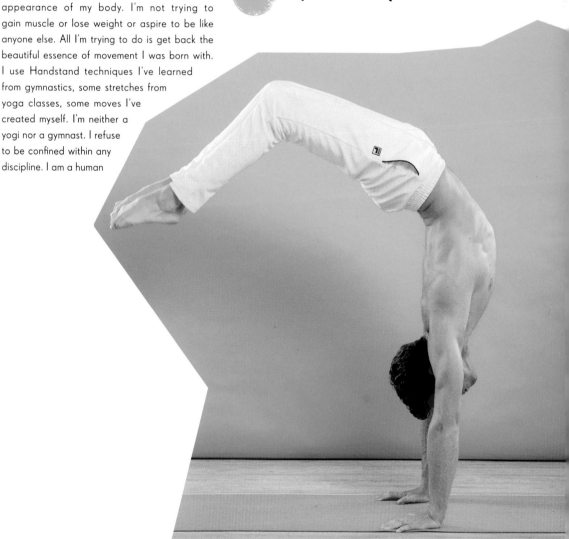

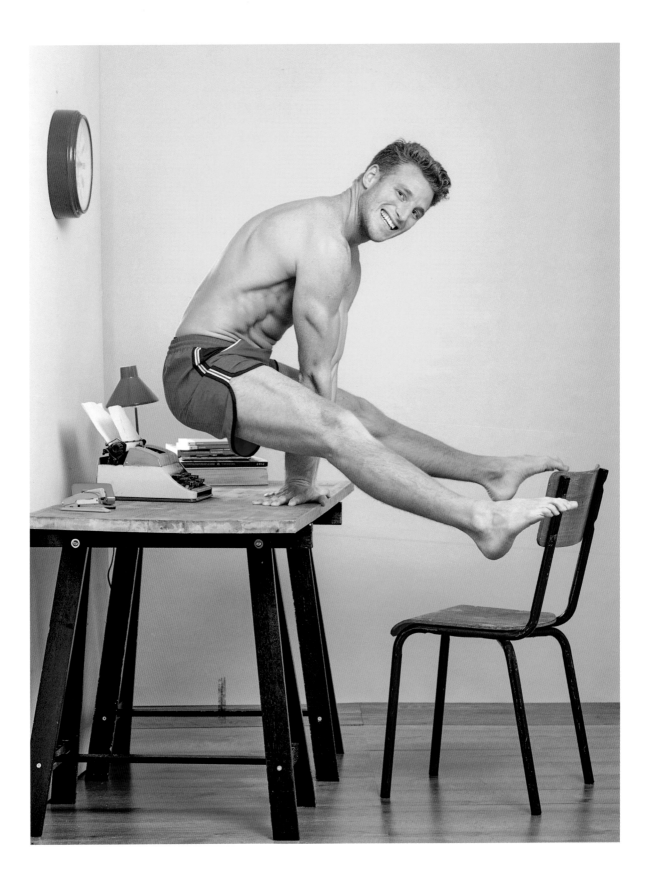

MOVEMENT FIRST

We've just learned what it means to be conscious in a movement, so now I want to explain about the "movement first" philosophy.

Okay, so stand up right now wherever you are with your feet together and your legs straight. Now press your heels against each other. I want you to notice what happened as a result of this movement. Did you feel that your butt muscles engaged? If you're pressing your heels together, it's impossible to avoid the muscular contraction in the butt that follows. Muscles engage as a result of a movement. This removes the need to focus on muscle engagement and encourages you to be more conscious of specific movements, because *movement comes first*. Here's the sequence:

Brain makes decision to move

Human moves

Hundreds of muscles in the body shift around to facilitate the movement

You see the whole body is interconnected.

THE BORING SCIENCE BIT

I really don't like to use jargon because:

1. It's theoretical and changes all the time.
2. I'm not a scientist. I simply look at the mechanics of how we were born to move.
3. We all moved perfectly before we even understood words, let alone scientific concepts.

My biggest belief is that we should all stop using jargon and start learning to move like we once could.

Sitting down for long periods of time freezes the spine into a constant flexed (rounded) position, putting repeated pressure on the same vertebrae.

As you freeze the range of motion in your legs, hips and spine, your body is left feeling tight and restricted, while your newly developed curved spine forces you to look down and literally makes you feel low. The curved spine shape also shrinks the space in which your lungs allow you to breathe, which may explain why you're suddenly out of breath when climbing a single flight of stairs. This reduction in oxygen entering your blood stream results in reduced concentration and alertness.

Repeated sitting also blocks fat-burning enzymes, stopping you from losing excess weight easily. No wonder those fitness programmes are failing!

You see, everything is made easier for us when we're older. We have priority seats on public transport, walking sticks, bungalows and stair lifts waiting for us to retire. Some of the biggest geriatric illnesses include: **coronary heart disease, stroke, respiratory diseases, metabolic dysfunction, type 2 diabetes.** And here is a separate list of the top diseases caused (in part) by a sedentary lifestyle: **coronary heart disease, stroke, respiratory diseases, metabolic dysfunction, type 2 diabetes.**
Did you notice anything similar about the last two lists? They are exactly the same.

In fact, at 75 years old, two-thirds of us will be suffering from a chronic illness and may be reliant on pharmaceutical treatment to keep us alive. However, this is "preventable" and in this book I'm not just going to teach you to "move". I'm going to teach you how to move like you were born to move.

A, B, C, D, E OF LONGEVITY

I promise, if you take the time to read through these next few pages before you start flicking through the rest of the book and attempting the exercises, you'll have a much better understating of what it takes to maintain a healthy body for the rest of your life. Plus, you might learn a few new things about your body.

A. A new language

B. Being aware of feelings

C. Comparing good feeling to pain

D. Defining the intensity

E. Enabling distractions

A NEW LANGUAGE

If you've ever had a conversation with, or worked alongside, a fitness professional – personal trainer, yoga teacher, physiotherapist – you may have noticed that they speak a specific language. They discuss the body from a theoretical perspective and give every twinge, restriction or inability a reason for what might be causing it. Their ideas seem plausible, but they live in a world of terminology and they talk the language of fitness. In this book, I deliver the language of human movement.

The language of movement gives you lifelong tools that you can use to derestrict your body. Anytime. Anywhere. For me, the process of derestricting should be available to all, a 70-year-old who is unable to leave the house as well as a 5-year-old in school. It is important to note that, as a two-year-old, you were capable of placing your elbows on the floor while sitting with your legs straight, but you'd never "stretched your hamstrings" to be able to do it. In fact, you couldn't even say the word "hamstrings". This language of fitness can inhibit your progress by telling you that there's something wrong with you when there isn't, like people being told they have flat feet or a weak core.

You see, as well as 800-odd muscles, humans are wrapped from head to toe in connective tissue. You may have heard of a thing called "fascia".

Many years ago, scientists discovered all the separate muscles in the body, named them and gave them responsibilities. The bicep is responsible for flexing the elbow, the tricep is responsible for extending the elbow and so on. It all made sense and they put all the information into a textbook with images of the muscles responsible for movement, giving exercises named after the muscles to strengthen and lengthen them: Lat Pull-down, Bicep Curl, Tricep Dip and so on.

But then we discovered fascia, a clingfilm-like substance that covers your body, from the top of your head to the soles of your feet. When we're born, the fascia in our bodies is supple, but as we become restricted, it can become tight and rigid. What I'm saying is that you can't move one part of your body without it having an effect on another, because fascia interconnects us... everywhere. The way I see it, we are one. A whole. A body.

So, let's get away from this theory of trying to improve muscles and look for something more tangible to improve, something that we can tell for ourselves. When we train, all that we feel is FEELING. I've said it before, but I'm going to say it again: your body is capable of billions – yes, billions – of movements. It's time to give up thinking about training muscles and get to the real issue: you have stopped moving naturally, and your first port of call is to regain that natural movement.

BEING AWARE OF FEELINGS

Have you ever looked at your dog or your cat, or in fact any animal, and said, "Oh, I wonder what they're thinking?" But they can't be, right? They don't have a language to think in. For us to even think that the dog is sitting there thinking is a bit ridiculous. Think about this.

If you didn't know language, you wouldn't be able to think either. You can't think in a language you can't speak. But would you still exist? Of course you would. As young children, we all existed without knowing language. Negativity, fear, stress, anxiety, worry, embarrassment, guilt, regret, sadness, bitterness, resentment. None of these existed for you then.

As a baby, when you needed a poo, you just had a poo. There was no voice in your head that said, "Oh my god, what will they think of me?" When you wanted something, you'd just cry. You enjoyed being out in the rain without using words like "miserable", and most importantly you existed – you just didn't have the access to language yet.

We could say that, at that time in your life, you were fully aware of what you were feeling because you weren't always in your head. You weren't thinking all the time.

When I was younger, I used to think I was different because I would talk to myself all the time. Now I realize that we all do! We have a constant internal dialogue that rarely switches off. The only problem with talking to yourself is that you are not being present in the moment and may become unaware of what's happening around you or what you are feeling. If you've ever meditated, you'll know the purpose of meditation is to watch your thoughts or to be aware that you're in a thinking state of mind.

So, how does this relate to the process of derestricting the body?

Have you recognized the feeling of being angry? When we get angry, we tend to say, "I am angry". You're not. You're Susan. You're Susan (or whatever your name is) naming the feeling that you call "anger". What is most important to understand is that when we are fully aware of ourselves (not always mindlessly thinking), we can become completely conscious of the feelings in our bodies.

What do you feel right now? Nothing? Then follow an exercise in this book to create a feeling. Becoming less controlled by your stream of thought and more aware of feelings in your body is not only one of the most powerful life tools that you will ever know, but will be extremely valuable in derestricting your body.

The more you become aware (conscious) of how your body feels at any given time, the better you'll become at recognising when to adjust your position in an exercise, which in turn will adjust the feeling. Awareness is everything. Think of this as your mantra:

"My body is not me, I am the watcher of my body. My job is to be conscious of and take care of my body until the very end."

COMPARING GOOD FEELING TO PAIN

Feelings, for each and every one of us, are unique and can only be defined by you, the feeler. I am the feeler of my feelings and you are the feeler of your feelings. I can have empathy, meaning I recognize that you are feeling a feeling, but I can't actually feel it for you. Once you understand this, the next thing you need to determine is the type of feeling that you are feeling.

If you've ever been through an upsetting break-up, you may describe that feeling as having your heart broken. Now, on a physical level, you're heart isn't actually broken, but that's what you feel.

When you pass your exams at school or get a promotion at work, you recognise a feeling of euphoria, pride, amazement, excitement, but in the same way as the example above, you may not go around physically jumping for joy yet you feel that type of feeling internally.

In these two examples, I used emotions to describe two different types of feeling. Now, I'm going to define the two different feelings that may occur in the process of derestricting your body.

The first is good feeling. Good feeling will feel like a stretchy or muscular sensation. I wouldn't describe it as a comfortable feeling, but as soon as you have found a feeling that feels uncomfortable, you can rest assured that you are derestricting your body or working for its greater good. In other words, if you feel a stretch or as if your muscles are burning, then something good is happening. This feeling is an indicator of progress. If you feel nothing, then nothing is happening. Simple as that.

All the time we're being sold comfort – a comfortable bed, sofa, car... But for the purpose of derestricting

your body, you've got to become good at being uncomfortable. However, don't confuse this with pain. You haven't got to get good at being in pain. That would be a bit ridiculous. Good feeling is not pain.

Pain is a feeling you are most likely to experience in your knees, elbows, shoulders, hips, neck, lower back or any area where bones are exposed. Most people will describe the feeling they feel as a harsh, acute or painful feeling. Every single one of us has experienced this. When the water tap runs too hot, you pull away. It's a signal – you're very clever body is sending you a message: "Don't go here!" It's telling you to stop. Pain, although not a nice feeling, is phenomenal, and the fact that you feel it means that your body is smart.

Nothing good will ever come of you being in physical pain. It's really not something I promote or advise people to persevere with.

In terms of derestricting your body, as soon as you feel pain, you need to stop what you're doing and find a good feeling by moving in a different way. Remember, we're looking for a feeling of discomfort, but never pain. You may need to go back several exercises in a move until you no longer feel pain.

The main reason I don't advise or teach fast movement is because of this warning pain. When you move fast, you miss the opportunity to feel what's happening in your body. It puts you in flight or fight mode, which produces hormones that mask these sensations. The slower you move, the more you can become aware of the different feelings in your body. Feelings are instant feedback on whether something is right and you should carry on, or wrong and you should stop.

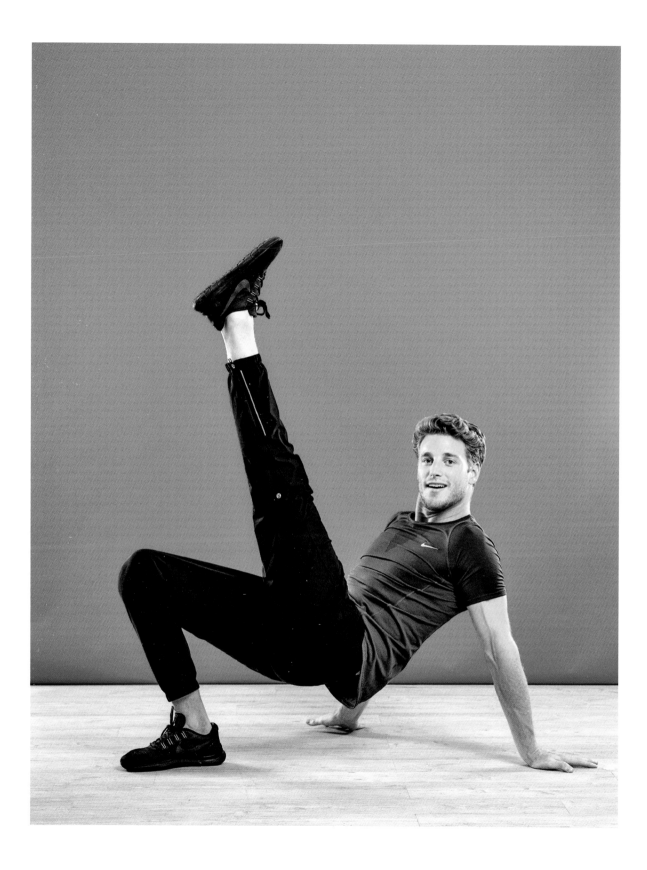

RESOLVING PAIN

The only way to find the solution to pain is to explore the sensation yourself. The second you go off looking for somebody to prod a thumb into your muscles, crack some bones or (worst of all) dampen down the sensation with some medication, you lose the opportunity to discover for yourself the root cause of the problem. So, no more external fixes. Next time, try this train of thought instead:

» Hmm... there is a sensation in my neck.
» What have I been doing lately that may have caused this sensation to arise?
» How many hours a day do I spend sitting on a chair or staring at a phone/computer screen?
» Do I actually have any awareness of how my body is moving throughout the day?
» When I do exercise, am I even conscious of how I move or do I just move?
» Do I get pumped up to exercise? (Being pumped up and moving fast can rob you of consciousness.)
» Am I prepared to take the time to learn where the restrictions are in my body and take action to do some long-term good?

DEFINING THE INTENSITY

For the purposes of derestricting the body, we need to be able to number the intensity we are feeling, and for this we use a simple scale of 1 to 10. So, if your boyfriend leaves the toilet seat up, how angry do you get? For some people 1; for others 10. Feelings are subjective to the feeler.

Years ago when I used to lift weights at the gym, I would always train to my maximum, and even when I couldn't do any more repetitions, I'd put all my effort into trying to get that bar to the top. Likewise, during my running days, I would summon every last ounce of power in me to cross the line in the quickest time. Then I got into yoga and I tried the same approach. Can you imagine how I looked putting all my energy into stretching? I'd cast my eyes around the room and see all the bendy people stretching and most seemed quite relaxed. I just put that down to, you know, once you get more flexible, it's easier. But that's not true – you just get better at coping with the feelings. When I started to relax a bit, my improvement went through the roof.

Based on the number system, when I first approached yoga, we could say I was using 10/10 effort.

So, if 10 is me in the stretch treating it like I need to cross the finish line as soon as possible, then the opposite of that is all you Child's Posers. Oh yeah, you know who you are: "I'm gonna chill here in my Child's Pose" or "I'm gonna do the least amount of effort until the teacher sees and then I'll work really hard for a few seconds before going back to my Child's Pose."

When trying to improve your movement, the ideal numbers to be working in are between 6 and 8, maybe 9 as you get better at coping with discomfort. 10 is too much; you're working too hard to be aware of what you feel and you'll end up injuring yourself. And if you're a 1, you might as well be sitting at home watching TV.

In A–D, we've learned that what we feel is unique feeling, that we can learn to be more conscious of our feelings, the difference between "good feeling" and "pain" and, lastly, how to number the sensations that we feel. Throughout the book, following the support exercises for each move, you will have the chance to test this effort scale on your body, but first we're going to learn one last thing, the power of distraction.

ENABLING DISTRACTIONS

Now, for the last step towards derestricting the body: the art of distraction.

Blink!

Because I just mentioned the word "blink", are you now aware that you are blinking? Were you aware of blinking previously?

Earlier, we discussed how feeling a good feeling may not be comfortable, but we know that it is a very necessary process if we want to derestrict our bodies. What we can do is exploit the fact that our minds are only capable of feeling one feeling at one time, or focusing on one thing at one time.

Look, you can't feel positive at the same time as feeling negative. You can't feel happy and sad together. They are complete opposites.

The benefit of only being able to feel one feeling at one time is the ability to distract yourself from uncomfortable feelings when in the process of derestricting your body.

Nobody in their right mind goes into a stretch and thinks, "Woo hoo, this feels so great, I want to do this all day long!" It can become an addictive thing and you might end up enjoying the feeling, but the real reward comes in the long term. You feel rewarded for doing it immediately and, more than that, you will start to see the reward in how your body moves.

To help with progress, you can distract yourself in any of the following ways, but you must always have an awareness of the feeling you feel in the background. You can:

» Focus purely on your breathing
» Watch TV
» Listen to music
» Dream of sitting on a beach
» Smile
» If you're outside, you can count the leaves on the trees

And that's my A–E of Longevity.

Derestricting the body is a lifelong process. It never stops. When you stop training your body to move, you give up responsibility for its health.

In movement, there is no alignment or perfect form. There is just feeling. The feeling you feel holds the key to where you are restricted and what action you need to take.

The question, "Where am I supposed to be feeling it?" is irrelevant. You should instead ask, "Where am I feeling it?" or "What feeling do I feel in my body right now?"

The steps I have shown you here are tools that you can use to get the job done. Nobody else can derestrict your body for you. Your personal trainer or yoga teacher cannot derestrict your body. They can of course give guidance and feedback, but nobody else can ever feel what you feel.

Don't think you're going to achieve the perfect, injury- and pain-free body – the one that sits in a squat, and can fold over at the waist with palms flat on the floor – in, let's say, six weeks.

Remember, the Frampton Method doesn't work on time restraints. You are designed to move well for the rest of your life. As soon as you give up movement, you give up on life. Your body will only do as much as you allow it to. You don't need to beat your body up, but you do need to be consistent. Movement is a habit that you must never ever forget again.

Go one step at a time, slowly, consciously. Remember that you're undoing years and years of damage. It takes time to remind your body of all the things it used to be able to do naturally and you have to be patient. I can assure you, though, it will come.

The hare game is finished – the tortoise wins this race.

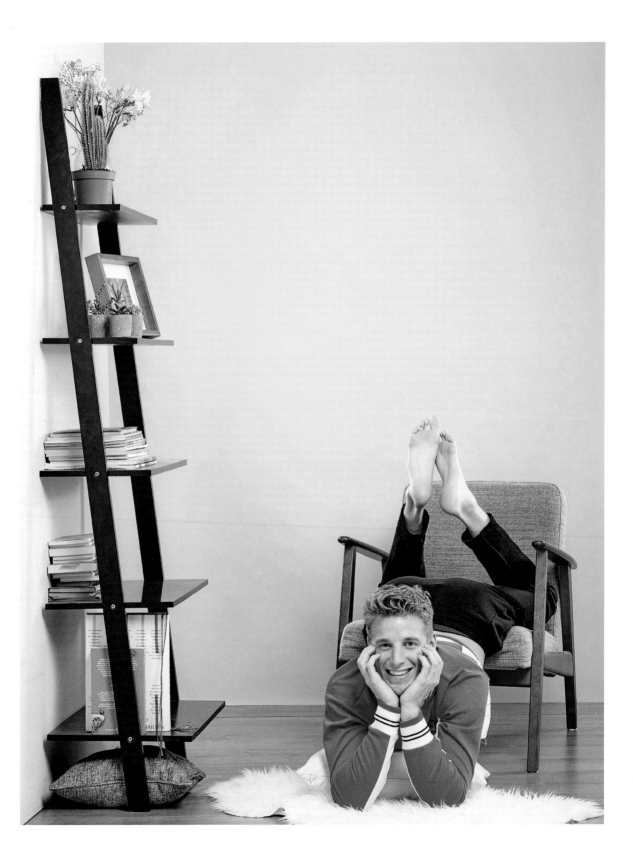

THE FRAMPTON PHRASEBOOK

Here's the list of terminology I'll be using throughout the book. It's important that you read this to understand the concepts otherwise it's highly likely you may get a little lost.

MOVEMENT Quite simply this is the exercise you are practising. That is all it is. If I use the word fitness, you might think I mean weight loss, a "leg day", workouts, cardio. I'm not referring to any of this. As I've said before, four-year-olds don't need these labels, and seeing as we're aiming to move like a four-year-old, neither do we. You were born with a perfect body and your goal is to use movement to regain and then maintain that body.

CONSCIOUSNESS This is your complete focus and awareness. Training with a watchful eye will catch the body out when it slips into a painful or harmful pattern of movement. Consciousness makes sure you make adjustments to correct yourself.

SENSATION This is the feeling that you feel when you are doing any movement. You need to be present, conscious, mindful and alert to feel individual sensations. When you've felt it, you have to label it mentally – identify it as good feeling or compensation (pain).

COMPENSATION (PAIN) Compensation is a painful feeling you're most likely to experience in your knees, elbows, shoulders, hips, neck or lower back – the bony bits. You might, for example, feel a pain in your lower back when you do a Bridge exercise – as an example, the compensation could be a result of having tight shoulders or it could be from having tight hips or in fact any restriction elsewhere in the body. Where the restriction occurs isn't important. What's important to grasp is that what you're feeling is a result of something else not moving as intended – that is, a compensation. Most people describe compensation as a harsh pain that sends the message, "Don't go here!" It's telling you to stop. Nothing good will ever come of you working into this painful sensation, but please don't get the wrong message that the sensation is bad. It's just a warning. As soon as you feel it, pause. If you feel pain in your knees when you squat, change the movement until you find good feeling or no pain. You may need to change the movement several times.

GOOD FEELING This is the feeling most of us feel down the back of our legs when we keep our legs straight and try to touch our toes. It's usually a muscular sensation that seems to stop you from going any further. Although uncomfortable, it is beneficial for long-term improvement. You will also come across good feeling when doing, say, the Front Support. This is a feeling that most will describe as a burning or fatiguing sensation. Again, although uncomfortable, a conscious burning sensation is necessary for long-term improvement.

RESTRICTION This is an area of the body that has become tight over a period of time. In order to survive, the human species has to adapt. In the process, we lose functions that we no longer need. In terms of movement, if you persistently use a chair rather than the natural squatting position, your body will lose access to the squat. As kids we could all bend over, legs straight, and place our palms on the floor, but now most of us can no longer even touch our toes. The body has shut down what it's not using. That's restriction.

In my opinion, there are three main culprits when it comes to restriction: shoes and tight clothing, chairs and screens. In turn, being restricted in movement causes four main problems: weight gain and even obesity (owing to lack of efficient output); lack of mobility, flexibility and strength; poor posture, injuries and pain; depression or a lack of self-worth.

However, remember that the solution to restriction is not to *move more*; it's to strip back and learn (or relearn) how to *move like we used to*. To do this, you'll hear me talk about "derestriction". Don't worry, I'm not going to ask you to start walking around in bare feet, loose clothing and quit your job to squat in public like a four-year-old. You're just going to learn where you have become restricted.

NEURAL PATHWAY Do you remember learning to stand up? Don't worry if you don't. For the majority of us this was a thing that took months and months of practise before we could stand without thinking abut it. The neural pathway I sometimes refer to in this book is essentially the connection between the brain and the body during a specific movement. Some people call this "muscle memory". Like learning to stand, crawl and walk, the movements in this book need to be learned. The best things take time!

THE

MOVES

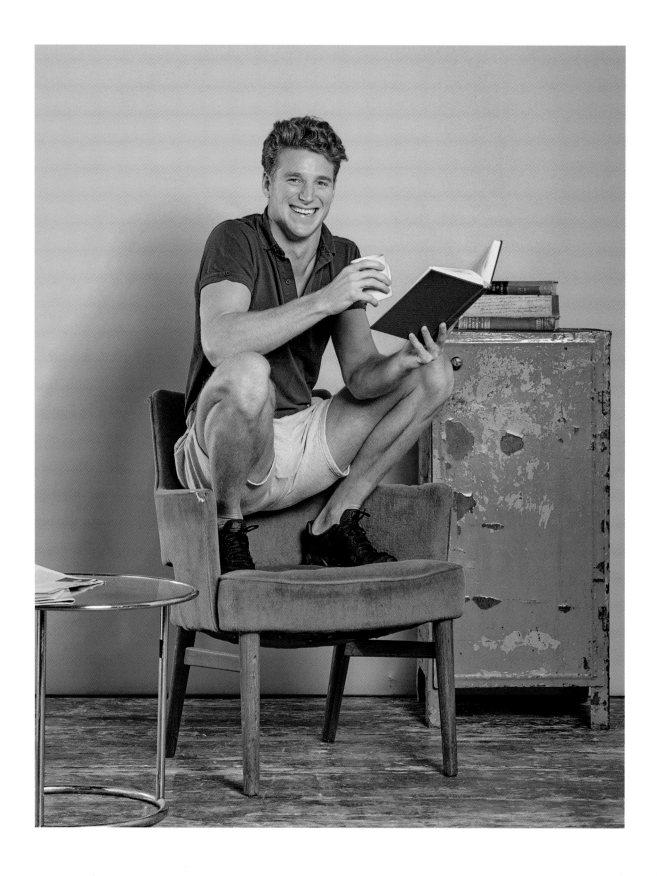

OVERHEAD SQUAT

The Squat is a very natural position, and was really simple... when you were four years old. If you have kids, or you have a friend that has kids, you will notice that those kids spend a lot of time sitting in a squat position. For kids, the Squat is not an exercise but a resting position.

However, when you were a kid, you were probably told to sit in a chair for everything: sit at the table to eat or to do your homework; sit on the sofa to watch TV. As soon as you started school, you were introduced into a day that included five hours of sitting. By the time you got to adulthood, sitting in a chair had become your default resting position. We're heading into the biggest epidemic of all time.

A study in 2012 found that musculoskeletal conditions were the second greatest cause of disability in the world, affecting more than 1.7 billion people worldwide. Professor Woolf, a world leader in healthcare, describes suffering from musculoskeletal disorders as being like a Ferrari without wheels: "If you don't have mobility and dexterity, it doesn't matter how healthy the rest of your body is."

We are all born with perfectly formed hips and spine, and it's high time to get our bodies back moving like they are designed to. Now, I'm not prepared to throw out a problem without providing you with a decent solution. Here goes...

BENEFITS
» Improved hip mobility
» Improved ankle mobility
» Improved body function
» Better awareness

But the biggest benefit of all: the squat is the position from which you can learn about the range of motion you have in the rest of your body. When you're in a squat position, it's very easy to recognise where other parts of your body have become restricted.

HOW TO MOVE
Choose 5 exercises from this book for your 10-minutes-a-day training. Identify the exercise in this section that you need to improve and repeat until you are able to progress to the next exercise. One exercise comprises both a 1-minute slow movement and a 1-minute static hold.

1. FOOT POSITION

First, we want to make sure our squat journey is injury free. When you're in the squat, the only part of your body in contact with the floor's surface is your feet. If you spend some time focusing on getting your foot position right, and build up from this, the journey to the full squat will be a simple and safe one.

Your feet should face forwards, *not* inwards and *not* outwards, and your forwards-facing feet should be arched.

Ever heard of flat feet? Perhaps somebody once told you that you are flat-footed? It could be that the shoes you've been wearing for the last few decades have caused your feet to lose their natural arched position and become flat. Well, you'll be pleased to know that your foot position is trainable.

A person once told me, "My feet turn out when I walk." My reply: "Stop allowing your feet to turn out when you walk." It sounds so simple, but when you become conscious of the way you stand, walk, squat and, most importantly, *move*, you can begin to change bad habits into good ones that keep you moving injury free. I mean, really, who controls your feet? You do. So, when you walk down the street, take responsibility for the way you move.

The first thing you need to do is stand up and look down at your feet. Next, face them forwards. For the squat, at no point will they need to turn outwards.

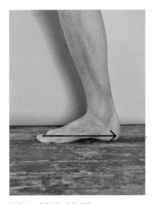
COLLAPSED FOOT

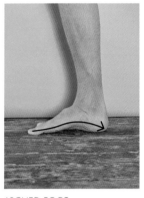
ARCHED FOOT

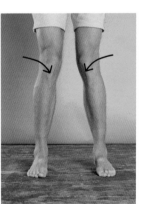
COLLAPSED FOOT

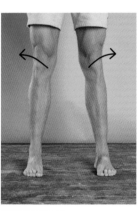
ARCHED FOOT

1-MINUTE MOVEMENT

Stand up and face your feet forwards, then **roll them between a collapsed position and an arched position,** using as wide a range of motion as you can. It will look something like the photos on the left.

1-MINUTE HOLD

Stay standing with your feet facing forwards and **roll your feet to an arched position,** keeping your big toe connected to the ground. Hold.

TIP: You'll notice that when the arches of your feet collapse, your knees turn inwards; when your feet are in an arched position, your knees rotate outwards.

2. ANKLE MOBILITY

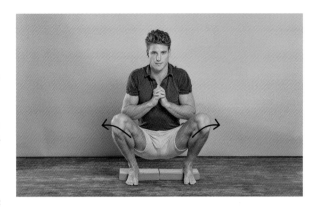

You're now going to repeat exactly the same movement as Exercise 1, only this time you're going to attempt it sitting in a squat position.

IMPORTANT: The higher the surface onto which you place your heels, the easier the movement will be. Using blocks to position your heels allows you to move easily without any pain at all.

1-MINUTE MOVEMENT

Move slowly between an arched foot and a collapsed foot while sitting in the squat position, elbows on thighs, hands clasped together. Focus on the following points:

» Feet face forwards
» Weight stays on the heels

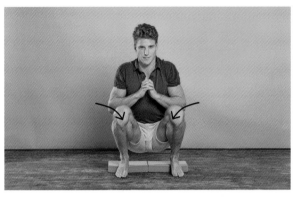

REMEMBER: When your knees are wide, your foot is in an arched position. When your knees come towards each other, your foot is in a collapsed position. Your toes should never leave the ground.

1-MINUTE HOLD

Hold your knees wide in an arched-foot position, as in the top photo. If you're doing this correctly, you should feel muscular tension on the outside of your hips around the butt area.

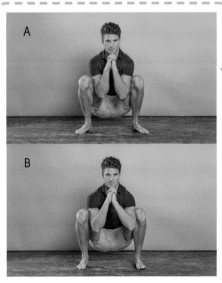

FOOD FOR THOUGHT

If you're wondering why we keep the feet facing forwards instead of turned out, as is commonly taught in yoga, there are two reasons:

» 1. Turning the feet out increases the risk of collapsed feet and long-term ankle and knee damage. The goal of a movement prioritises the long-term benefits for your body.
» 2. Keeping the feet facing forwards ensures you maximise the effects of flexibility of your hips, rather than resting on the joint.

Let's play a game to check that you're staying on track. One of the images above is incorrect and one is correct. Which is the correct one?

Answer: B is correct, feet facing forwards.

3. SPINE ROLL ON BLOCK

For Exercise 3, you're going to focus your attention on the movement of your spine in the squat. You'll need to keep your feet facing forwards while your attention goes elsewhere.

In the left photo, I am taking my spine to the most flexed position I can. In the right photo, I have lifted my spine into the most extended position I can.

Ask someone to take a photograph of you in this position, or use a mirror to see what your spine looks like. A good way to know you're in a fully extended position is to see if you're able to rest your elbows on top of your knees.

1-MINUTE MOVEMENT
Squat on a block (or blocks – use as many as you need to) and roll your spine from a flexed to an extended position. Aim to sit your elbows on top of your knees. If this means shrugging your shoulders, raise your heels using more blocks until you can do it without a shrug.

The photographs at the bottom of the page show my elbows too far forwards, and too far back with my shoulders shrugged.

1-MINUTE HOLD
Squat on a block (or blocks), **hold your elbows on top of your knees and extend your spine**. Remember all the points so far:
» Feet facing forwards
» Feet in the arched position
» Elbows on top of knees
» Shoulders relaxed (not shrugged up around your ears)

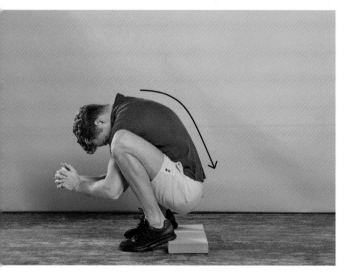
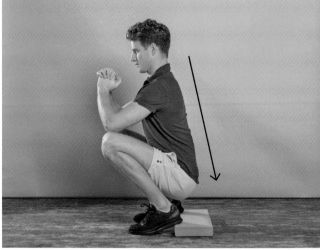

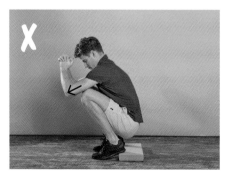
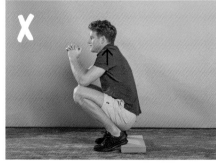

4. ANKLE MOVEMENT USING SUPPORT

For Exercise 4, you're going to sit in the squat on a flat surface, but holding onto something for support. Use something like a lamppost, a bar or a sturdy chair – anything that counterbalances your weight.

This is the first exercise in which your heels will be in full contact with the floor. If you feel any joint pain (you might feel it in your knees), keep practising pain-free Exercise 3, until you can achieve the position of Exercise 4 without discomfort.

1-MINUTE MOVEMENT

Use the movements from Exercises 1 and 2 (see pages 34–35), but this time with your support fully supporting your weight so that you can focus fully on the movement of your feet rather than worrying about toppling over: **roll your feet from a collapsed to an arched position**. *Do not* lift up onto your toes. Your weight must remain on your heels with your toes in contact with the floor.

1-MINUTE HOLD

Your aim here is to **hold your feet in the arched position with your knees as wide as possible**. Keep your feet facing forwards at all times. You should start to feel a burning sensation around your butt area and the outsides of your hips. You may also feel that sense of burning (a muscular sensation that indications good feeling; see below) inside your hips and your shins. This is perfectly normal – as long as you don't feel pain, hold the position.

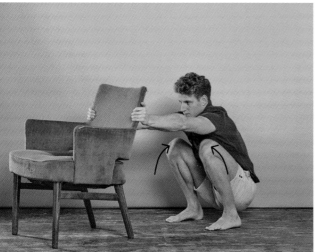
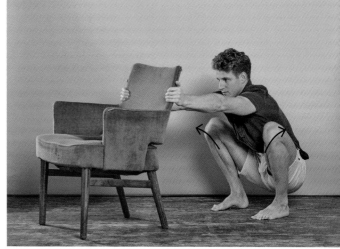

FOOD FOR THOUGHT

Good feeling is a muscular sensation. I wouldn't describe it as pleasant, but it *is* beneficial, as it contributes to the long-term benefit of exercise for your body. *Bad pain*, on the other hand, is not effective for the long-term benefit of your body.

5. SUPPORTED SPINE ROLL

In Exercise 5, you're going to practise the spine roll from Exercise 3, only this time using a support. You aren't using the block and are sitting fully in the squat on a flat surface. This exercise will also introduce you to a straight-arm movement that will come up throughout the book.

In this exercise, you'll learn to hold yourself in an upright position using your core rather than gripping with your arms. You may find that you need to move closer or further away from your support until you find a spot that is comfortable for you.

1-MINUTE MOVEMENT

Sit in the squat on a flat surface, holding onto your support and keeping the weight on your heels. **Move between a flexed or rounded spine and an extended or straight spine position**. In the flexed-spine position, your knees should be under your armpits; in the extended-spine position, your chest should come away from your knees.

1-MINUTE HOLD

Sit in the squat on a flat surface, holding onto your support and keeping the weight on your heels. **Hold your body in the extended-spine position**. Keep your arms straight.

Remember all the points so far:
» Feet facing forwards on a flat surface
» Use your support to remain stable
» Weight on your heels
» Arms straight
» Chest away from knees
» Shoulders in a relaxed position – *not* shrugged

TIP: Focus on pushing your shoulders back and down at the top of the position to help keep your spine extended and to prevent any shrugging.

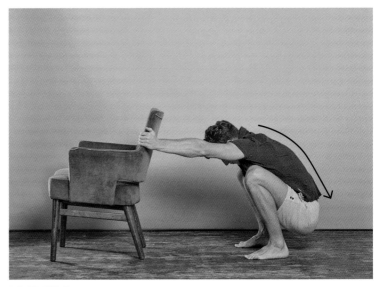

FLEXED SPINE

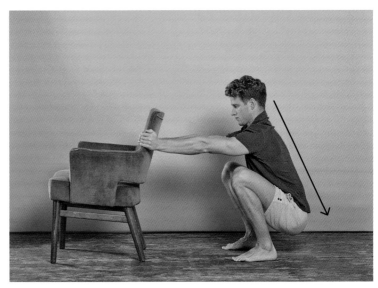

EXTENDED SPINE

6. BLOCK HEAD

Exercise 6 is a movement that can be effective for opening up the hips (which in turn can help you to achieve the full squat position). You'll need your blocks – the higher you place them in front of you, the easier the exercise.

You may not feel tightness here at all. I've taught people who can barely sit in a crossed-legged position, and I've also taught people who can sit very comfortably crossed-legged with their head resting on the floor and feel no stretch whatsoever. Every body is unique. If you feel no stretch as you practise this exercise, skip to Exercise 7. If you feel some tightness (a restriction), stick with it.

NOTE: Restriction is an area of the body that has become tight over time.

1-MINUTE MOVEMENT

Sit upright in a crossed-legged position with a block in front of you. Upend the block for the least stretch, place it on its side for a medium stretch and flat for the furthest stretch – use whichever is pain free. **Reach your head forwards, bending from the hips, until you touch the block with your forehead.**

Raise up to the start position, then lower again, changing the position of the block as the sensation (stretch) dissipates. Cross your legs the other way and repeat to work different areas of the body.

Your elbows will lower towards the floor in front of your knees as you bend. As the sensation dissipates, you'll be able to get lower and lower until one day you can rest your head on the floor with no blocks at all.

IMPORTANT: You should feel no pain in your knees. If you do, position your feet further away from your body.

1-MINUTE HOLD

Sit cross-legged. **Rest your head on the block with your elbows on the floor and hold.** Swap the cross. As you regain flexibility and the sensation dissipates, drop the blocks until your head meets the floor.

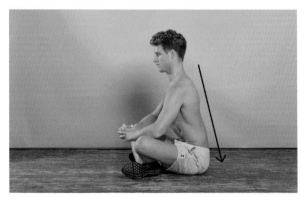
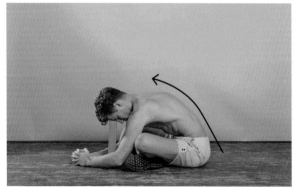
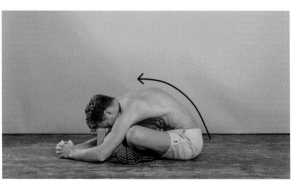
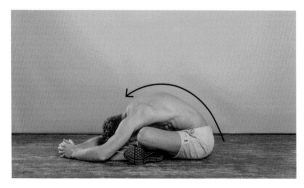

7. WIDE KNEES ("THE FROG")

Exercise 7 looks for restrictions in the insides of the legs, around your groin area. You'll need to place each of your knees on a block with your hips directly above or ideally behind your knees towards your feet. Use a mirror or ask someone to take a photograph of you.

Your shins should be parallel to one another and at right angles to your thighs. The priority is to keep your hips in line with your knees. The aim is to move backwards towards your heels.

1-MINUTE MOVEMENT

Adopt the position described above. **Move slowly between an untucked pelvis and a tucked pelvis**, while keeping your knees and hips square to each other. In an untucked pelvis position, you should have a slight dip in your lower back. In a tucked pelvis position, you should have a flat back.

Tap into the sensations. Are they good or bad (see page 37)? How intense are they, on a scale of 1 to 10?

1: "I could sit here all day long." (This is not enough for long-term improvement.)

10: "I need to stop *now*!" (Be patient: work towards long-term improvement, moving down the scale.)

Don't be lazy and don't go crazy: aim for a 7 or 8.

1-MINUTE HOLD

Hold the tucked pelvis position, numbering the sensation – if it is higher than 8, bring your knees towards each other; if it is lower than 7, slide your knees apart. Focus on the following:

» Hips above knees or slightly behind
» Shins parallel and at right angles
» Elbows on the floor

TOP UNTUCKED PELVIS
BOTTOM TUCKED PELVIS

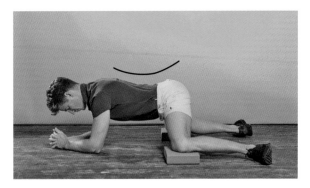

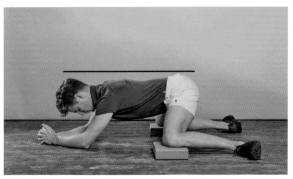

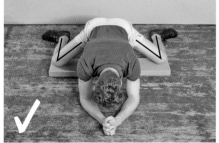

PARALLEL ALIGNMENT

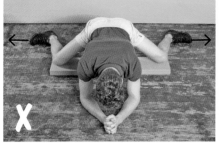

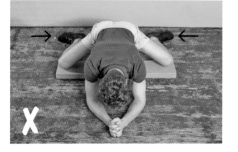

10

9

8

7

6

5

4

3

2

1

8. SPINE ROLL ON FLOOR

For Exercise 8, you're coming back to the squat position. You'll need to be completely comfortable sitting in a full squat on a flat surface – if you're unable to do this yet, do the exercise with blocks under your heels, then over time remove the blocks until you're able to do it without.

1-MINUTE MOVEMENT

Starting in a full squat with your feet shoulder-width apart, **roll your spine from a flexed position (with your body between your knees, hands clasped) to an extended position (chest pulled away)**. At the top of the movement, the goal is to place your elbows on top of your knees with your palms together, fingers clasped.

1-MINUTE HOLD

Sit in a full squat, elbows on top of your knees, spine extended. Remember to keep your shoulders relaxed. Focus on the following:

- » Feet shoulder-width apart
- » Feet facing forwards
- » Weight on heels
- » Elbows on knees
- » Palms together
- » Chest upright
- » Look straight ahead
- » Shoulders back and down

IMPORTANT: For this exercise I am wearing footwear with a low heel. If your shoes have a heel, switch to bare feet or wear footwear that keeps your heels as low to the floor as possible.

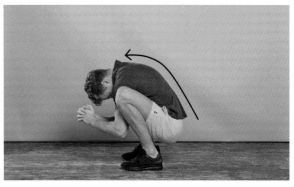

FLEXED SPINE (BODY BETWEEN KNEES)

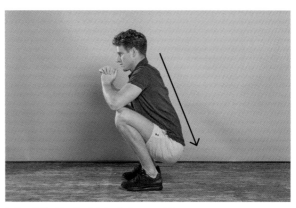

EXTENDED SPINE (ELBOWS ON KNEES)

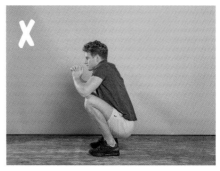

Remember, don't shrug.

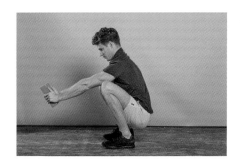

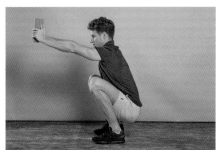

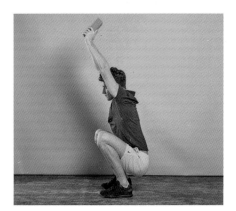

1-MINUTE MOVEMENT

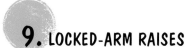

9. LOCKED-ARM RAISES

For Exercise 9, you're staying in the full squat, but moving on to develop the straight-arm work that we touched on in Exercise 5, this time using a block. When you come to do the Front Support (see pages 44–55), you'll need to have learned this technique to press through your shoulders.

NOTE: Don't just hold the block – actively press it up and away from you, even it moves only a tiny bit.

1-MINUTE MOVEMENT

Sit fully in the squat position and **press the block away from you,** keeping your elbows locked (left, top photo). Once you can fully lock your arms, **raise the block as high as possible, pressing it away and up until it is above your head** (left, bottom photo).

1-MINUTE HOLD

Sit fully in the squat position. **Hold the block as far up and back as possible, sliding your shoulder blades up your back to do so** (below, second from left photo). Keep your hips low, taking care that they do not raise up and away from the ground. Make sure you don't squeeze your back muscles up into your neck. Take a look at the correct and incorrect photographs (below). Keep going through the following points:

» Feet facing forwards
» Knees wider than hips
» Elbows locked
» Block pressed up and away using your back muscles (not your neck)
» Shoulder blades slide up the back

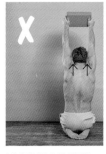

MUSCLES SQUEEZE
INTO NECK

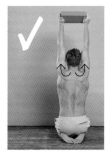

SHOULDER BLADES
SLIDE UPWARDS

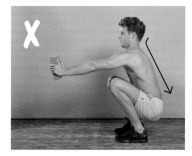

DON'T EXTEND YOUR NECK

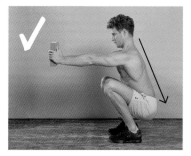

LET YOUR ARMS LEAD THE MOVEMENT

10. LOWERING INTO SQUAT WITH ARMS OVERHEAD

For Exercise 10, the objective is to start from a standing position facing a wall and lower into the squat position without letting the block touch the wall.

1-MINUTE MOVEMENT

Stand with your feet facing forwards and your knees wider than your hips. **Press the block up and overhead, and at the same time, slowly lower straight down to your lowest squat**. The aim is to *slowly* **lower all the way to the bottom and back up again** without the block touching the wall, retaining the positions of your feet and hips.

1-MINUTE HOLD

Stand facing a wall, feet facing forwards and shoulder-width apart. Position yourself as close to the wall as possible so that you can **squat with the block overhead, but without letting it touch the wall** as you lower. Hold the lowest position.

NOTE: As you improve, move closer to the wall, until one day your toes actually touch it when you lower.

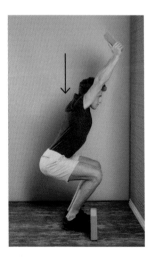
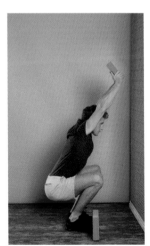

LIFE HACKS

TRAINSQUATTING

You can practise your moves anytime, anywhere – whenever you have a spare minute or some dead time. Imagine me on the train to work, checking my emails on my phone. Am I sat in a chair? No, I'm squatting. Not only do I avoid more chair-sitting, but I actually improve my squat position.

COMMUTER HOLD

I call this "secret stretching". For one train stop, sit in the squat position against a flat surface. As your flexibility improves, squat for more stops.

NOTE: Your lower back must be in contact with the surface behind you. Don't allow your pelvis to tuck under.

For more advice on how to do this, see www.roger.coach.

CONGRATULATIONS!

If you've mastered this move, you're now squatting like you could when you were a four-year-old. Don't ever let life take this position away from you again. And if you're now up for a bigger challenge, practise all the squat exercises (from 1 to 10) using only one leg. Good luck!

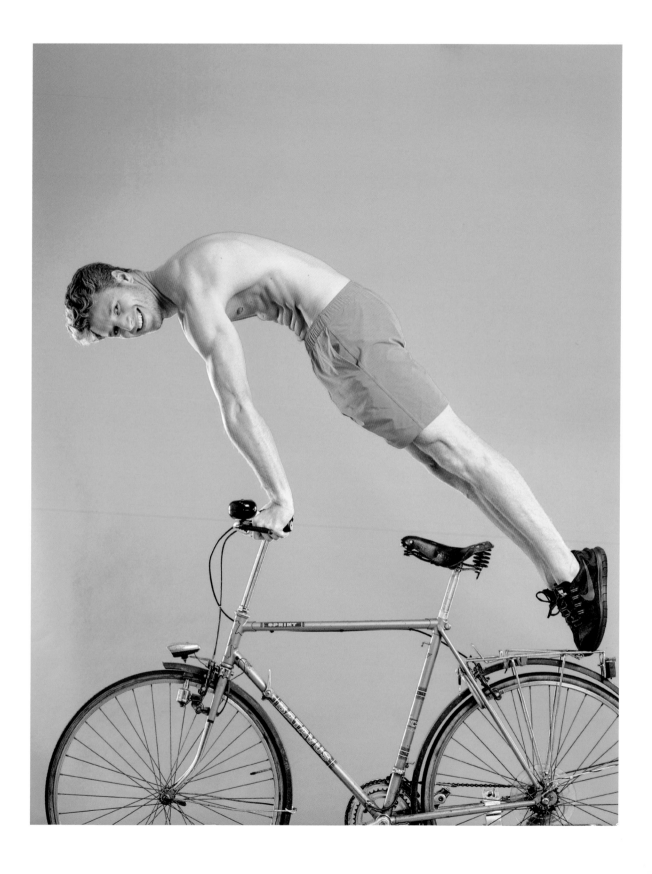

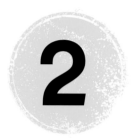

FRONT SUPPORT

The Plank is one of the most common exercises in the fitness industry today. At first glance, you may think that this move is just another plank. However, this is called the Front Support, an exercise Olympic gymnasts use as one of their routine strengthening body alignment exercises.

The Plank is well known as a core exercise, but the Front Support is a true test of how active your back and butt muscles are, as well as your core. In this chapter, I will explain how to hold a Front Support correctly, how to avoid pain and what common mistakes inhibit your progress.

With practice, you'll be able to hold the perfect Front Support with your palms pressing through the ground, your upper back rounded, shoulders pressing, rib cage pulled in, stomach sucked in, pelvis tucked under, knees locked and heels together. Sound like a lot to do? No problem. Let me show you how.

BENEFITS
» Improved butt muscles
» Improved pelvis mobility
» Awareness of your back muscles
» Improved spine alignment
» Core strength
» Shoulder strength
» Better awareness of your body

HOW TO MOVE
Choose 5 exercises from this book for your 10-minutes-a-day training. Identify the exercise in this section that you need to improve and repeat until you are able to progress to the next exercise. One exercise comprises both a 1-minute slow movement and a 1-minute static hold.

1. ARM LOCK

Exercise 1 teaches you the locked-arm position. It's the same arm movement used for pressing away the block in the Locked-Arm Raises (see page 42).

1-MINUTE MOVEMENT

Kneel on the floor, knees and thighs together, sitting back on your heels. Interlock your fingers, palms facing your body. **Press your hands away from you at shoulder height, until you go from a straight back to a rounded back.** Try to create as much distance as possible between your ribs and your hands. At the point where your arms are fully locked, three things will happen:

» Arms rotate so that your biceps face upwards
» Ribs suck in
» Upper back rounds so that your shoulder blades are no longer visible

Keep moving back and forth.

1-MINUTE HOLD

Adopt the starting position for the movement. **Press away your interlinked hands so that your back rounds.** Hold this position, making sure you keep your arms at shoulder height.

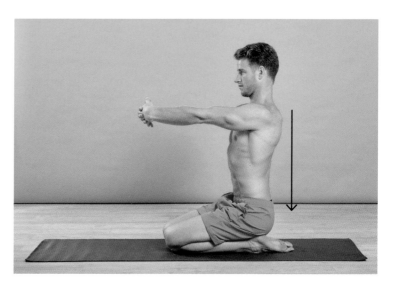

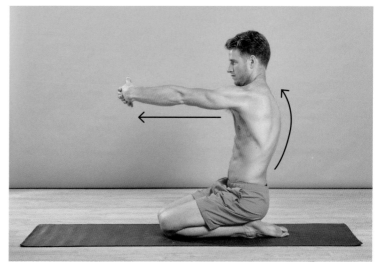

2. KNEELING LOCK

In Exercise 2, you're going to perform the same arm movement as Exercise 1. However, rather than sitting back on your knees, you're going to practise it on all fours on the floor. This is not a push-up; your arms do not bend. You're pushing with your shoulders to round your back.

1-MINUTE MOVEMENT

Kneel on the floor on all fours with your back straight and your hands beneath your shoulders, fingers pointing forwards. Keep your arms straight. **Move slowly, straightening your arms and rounding your shoulders and upper back.** Focus on sucking in your ribs, rotating your elbows to face behind you and pressing your hands into the floor. Your shoulders should stack directly above your hands, without hunching, and your eyes should be looking downwards.

1-MINUTE HOLD

From the starting position in the movement, **press through the floor to round your shoulders, pull your ribs in as much as you can and hold.** You should feel a burning sensation around your shoulders, back and arms.

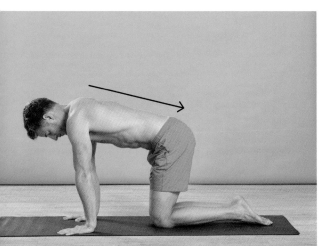

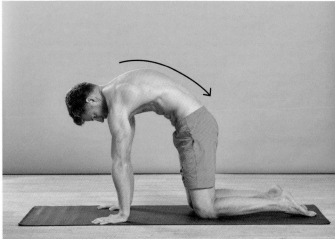

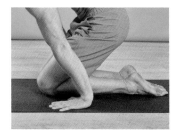

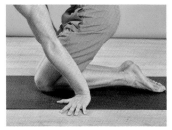

FOOD FOR THOUGHT

When I say "hands pressed into the floor", your fingers should point forwards and the underside of the knuckle of your index finger should stay connected with the floor (far left photo). If you feel pain in your wrists, turn your fingers out slightly (near left photo), but remember to always keep your index finger connected.

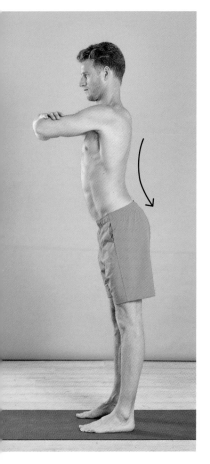
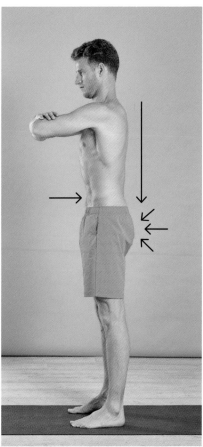

3. TUCKING THE PELVIS

For Exercise 3, you're going to get up to do a standing exercise. First, look at the photographs and focus on the differences between the look of an untucked and a tucked pelvis. Then, we'll move on to what they feel like.

1-MINUTE MOVEMENT

Stand straight, feet hip-width apart. **Raise your arms to shoulder height and fold them**. Untuck your pelvis and notice the arch in your back. Then, **engage your butt muscles to tuck in your pelvis**. Your back straightens. Move between tucking and untucking your pelvis for the full minute.

NOTE: Do not focus on your stomach muscles for this exercise; your butt muscles are the key. You can use your butt muscles to tuck in your pelvis, or you can tuck in your pelvis to engage your butt. I don't care which one you focus on just be completely clear at this stage which is which.

1-MINUTE HOLD

Begin in the standing position at the start of the movement. **Tuck in your pelvis, squeeze your butt and hold.**

4. KNEELING TUCK

The images below look exactly the same as the images in Exercise 2. However, this time you're going further down the chain to focus on the movement of your pelvis.

1-MINUTE MOVEMENT

Position yourself on all fours, as in Exercise 2 (see page 47). **Move between an arched back and a rounded back, and this time also use the tuck in your pelvis to make the switch**. At the very top of the movement, you should feel your butt muscles engage. At the same time, you will move from a flat to a rounded back, just as you did in Exercise 2.

1-MINUTE HOLD

You're now having to focus on several things at once. It's complex at first, and getting it right will take practice. Assume the starting position for the movement and **tuck in your pelvis, then hold**. Keep repeating the following in your head as you hold the position:

» Hands pressed into the floor
» Rounded upper back
» Arms locked and elbows rotated to face behind
» Ribs sucked in
» Eyes looking down and slightly in front of the hands
» Pelvis tucked under
» Butt muscles engaged

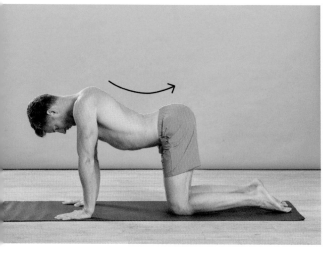
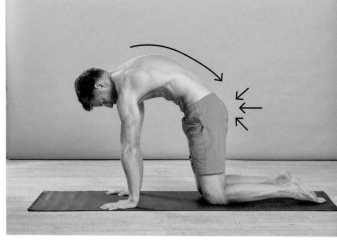

5. PISTOL SQUAT HOLDS

This exercise is for single leg-locking, which will fully engage the muscles around your knees.

1-MINUTE MOVEMENT
Build up your blocks or books underneath one of your heels until you can comfortably **raise and hold your other heel off the ground with your leg straight out in front of you, locking your knee. Move slowly, lowering and raising the extended leg.** Do this for 30 seconds each side, or spend longer on the side that feels harder.

1-MINUTE HOLD
Begin in the starting position for the movement, with one leg extended and your other heel on the block(s). **Raise the extended leg off the ground in a locked position.** Hold for 30 seconds, then repeat with the other leg.

NOTE: You may find this exercise easier on one side than the other. If so, work on the weaker side more, until it is equally easy on both sides.

If you're finding the Pistol Squat tricky, try the exercise on page 131.

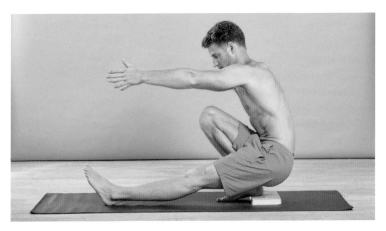

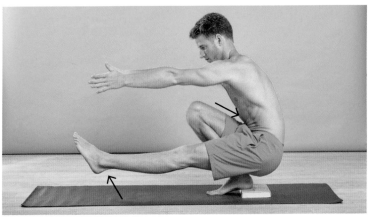

6. LEG LOCK IN FRONT SUPPORT

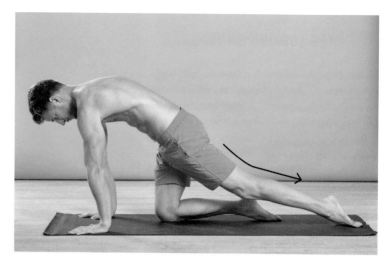

In the previous exercise, you familiarised yourself with what it feels like to lock your legs. The goal in Exercise 6 is to be able to extend and lock one leg in a Front Support position.

1-MINUTE MOVEMENT

Starting in the same position as Exercise 4 (see page 49), **extend one leg behind you and lock it completely**. Return to the starting position and then extend the opposite leg and lock it completely. Take turns with each leg for the full minute. You should feel the straight leg activate and the butt engage.

TIP: You can keep your foot pointed or flexed as feels more comfortable.

1-MINUTE HOLD

Hold the straight leg locked in position for 30 seconds, then repeat with the other leg.
Remember the following as you hold:
» Hands pressed into the floor
» Upper back rounded
» Arms locked and elbows rotated to face behind you
» Ribs sucked in
» Eyes looking down and slightly in front of your hands
» Pelvis tucked under
» Butt muscles engaged on the locked leg

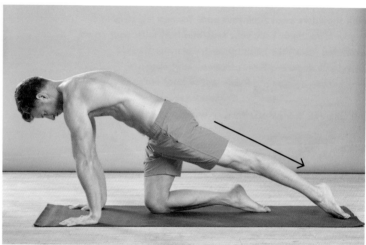

9. PELVIS-TUCKED-IN FRONT SUPPORT

For Exercise 9, the goal is to move from a tucked pelvis to an untucked pelvis while holding your legs in a locked position. Remember the movement in Exercise 3, where we were mastering a standing tuck (see page 48)? This is the upgraded version of that.

Ever heard of muscle memory? Well, I can assure you that muscles themselves *do not* have memory. However, movements *do*. Your goal is to rewire your brain so that it remembers how to move your body like it once could.

How it works is this: you train a movement in basic terms, rather like Exercise 1 (see page 46), focusing on one thing. By the time you've mastered Exercise 9, it's not the muscles that are remembering how to move, it's your brain registering hundreds of tiny movements. In other words, the more complicated the exercises become, the smarter and more body aware you become.

1-MINUTE MOVEMENT

Start in the hold position for Exercise 8 (see page 53), then lower so that you create a perfect line from your shoulder to your toes, as in a full Front Support. Staying in your line, **tuck in your pelvis to create a hollow in your back, then untuck, causing your upper back to round and your lower back to flatten**. Repeat for the full minute, without allowing your body to move up or down.

REMEMBER: As you tuck your pelvis in, you will feel your butt muscles engage; and you'll feel them release as you untuck.

1-MINUTE HOLD

Raise yourself into the Front Support position and tuck in your pelvis. Hold like this for the full minute.

FOOD FOR THOUGHT

In the photographs, I have pointed toes, but you may find it easier to raise yourself up onto flexed toes (toes under). We'll work on pointing the toes in the next exercise. For now, get used to pushing your heels against each other, which will further help you to feel your butt muscles engage.

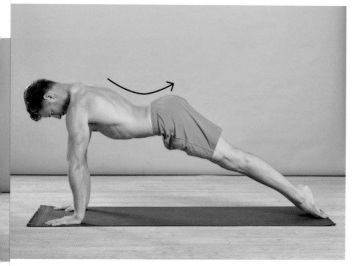
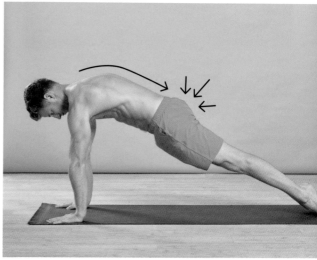

10. POINTED-TO-FLEXED IN YOUR LINE

Once you have mastered Exercise 9, you should be able to move slowly and consciously between pointed toes and flexed toes while you are holding the line of the Front Support.

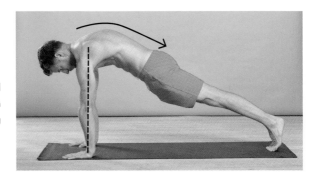

1-MINUTE MOVEMENT

Follow the instructions for the hold position in Exercise 9, only this time have your feet flexed. Tuck in your pelvis. **Rock forwards slightly, reducing the angle at your wrist, to move from a flexed-foot position to a pointed position,** while keeping the strong line of the Front Support. Rock back and forth like this for the full minute.

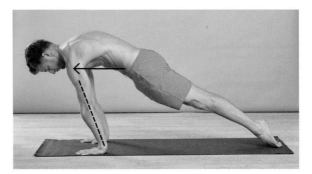

1-MINUTE HOLD

Begin in the **Front Support position with pointed toes**. Hold, focusing on the following:
» Hands pressing through the ground
» Arms locked and elbows rotated backwards
» Ribs pulled in
» Pelvis tucked
» Upper back rounded
» Butt muscles engaged
» Legs locked
» Heels together
» Toes pointed

CONGRATULATIONS!

You are now a master of the perfect Front Support (you can call it a Plank if you like). This is a foundation for your bodyweight work, because all the exercises you've mastered to get here will come up again throughout the book. And, if you're ready for something more challenging, come on over to the Headstand (see page 112) and hold a solid line with three – rather than four – points of contact. Good luck!

LIFE HACK

STANDING POSITION

Standing strong will not only give you better posture, burn more calories and potentially save you from joint replacements, but also help you become more bodily aware and more flexible.

A PLANK STAND?

A gymnastic Handstand, although a challenging exercise, puts the body through the same techniques as the perfect Front Support. Look at a gymnast doing a Handstand and consider:
» Hands pressing through the ground
» Arms locked
» Ribs pulled in
» Upper back rounded
» Pelvis tucked under
» Stomach sucked in
» Butt muscles engaged
» Legs locked
» Toes pointed
For more advice on how to do this, see www.roger.coach.

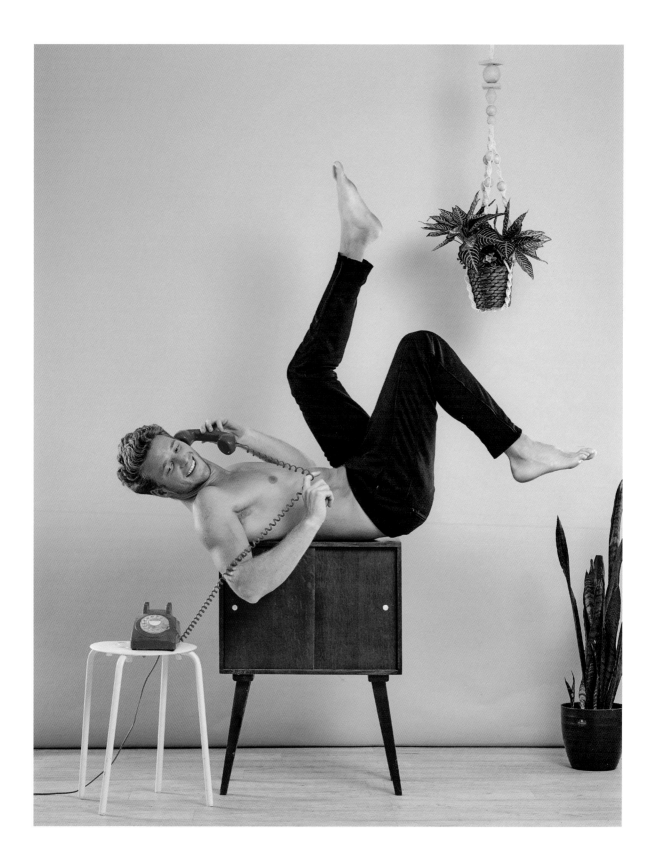

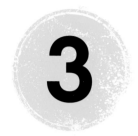

3

HOLLOW BODY

The Hollow Body is an exercise taken straight from gymnastics. Not only will this exercise teach you how to hold your body in a straight line, it will also highlight what areas of your body you need to work on: whether you have tight shoulders or tight hips, or need to boost your core strength, spine flexibility or even leg flexibility, this exercise will reveal all.

There are a number of things going on during this exercise, but if you follow the steps slowly and patiently, in addition to being able to perform the Hollow Body, you'll fully understand what your body is doing and what it can achieve.

You'll learn how to simultaneously keep your: stomach sucked in, arms locked, shoulders externally rotated (open), ribs pulled in and butt engaged.

BENEFITS
» Decrease in lower back pain
» Core strength
» Rib cage mobility
» Shoulder flexibility
» Hip flexibility
» Better awareness of your body
» Sets the foundation for the body-line to achieve the Headstand (see pages 112–127)

HOW TO MOVE
Choose 5 exercises from this book for your 10-minutes-a-day training. Identify the exercise in this section that you need to improve and repeat until you are able to progress to the next exercise. One exercise comprises both a 1-minute slow movement and a 1-minute static hold.

1. ROCKING TUCKS

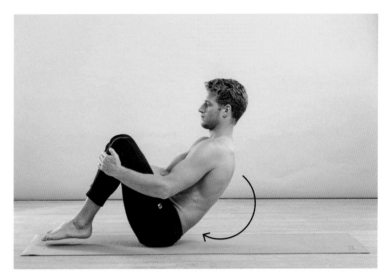

The objective of Exercise 1 is to get you used to having your spine in contact with a surface. It's a good warm-up exercise, too.

The most important point is to ensure you feel your lower back connect with the floor. As you make your way through the 10 exercises in this chapter, you'll find it increasingly challenging to make that brain-to-body connection. Take time to master now how your lower back connects with the floor, and you'll be less likely to lose the ability to notice it once you're incorporating more complicated moves.

1-MINUTE MOVEMENT

Sit down on a mat or soft surface with enough space behind you to roll backwards. Tuck your knees into your stomach and use your hands to hold them there; keep your feet flat on the floor. Then, **raise your feet and begin to roll backwards**, connecting every part of your spine with the floor as you do so, right to the top. Immediately, **roll forwards again until your feet touch the floor**. Roll backwards and forwards like this for 1 minute.

1-MINUTE HOLD

Lie down on a mat or soft surface and **bring your knees to your chest, curling yourself into a ball**. Your hips, head and shoulders will be off the ground, and your chin will be tucked into your chest. Hold. As you hold, notice your lower back press into the floor.

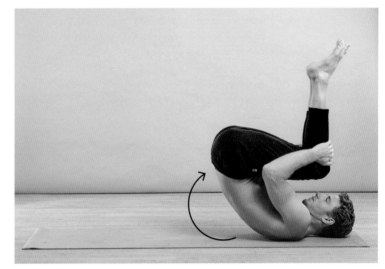

2. STOMACH CONTROL IN A HOLLOW TUCK

For Exercise 2, you're going to work on controlling your stomach muscles, which can be trained in two ways:

1. Squeezing the abdominals (external)
2. Sucking in the stomach (internal)

To master the Hollow Body, it's vital from the off that you spend some time understanding the difference between external and internal when it comes to your stomach. For the Hollow Body, the focus is sucking in (internal).

When you crunch (left photo) the distance between the base of your ribs and your belly button will reduce. Your upper back raises higher off the floor and your lower back presses down into the floor. This is **squeezing** the abdominals (external).

When you suck in and lengthen, lowering your upper back towards the floor (right photo), you increase the distance between the base of your ribs and your belly button. Your lower back stays in contact with the floor and your shoulders raise just off the floor. This is **sucking** the stomach in (internal).

In both movements, it is essential that your lower back remains in contact with the floor.

1-MINUTE MOVEMENT

Lie on your back on the floor, knees bent, feet off the floor, arms by your sides. **Slowly squeeze your abdominals to raise your upper back and shoulders, while keeping your knees tucked in. Lift your arms, too (left photo)**. When you've reached the top of the movement, **suck in your stomach and lower your spine to the floor, keeping your feet raised**. Move slowly back and forth between crunching the abdominals (external) and sucking the stomach in (internal).

1-MINUTE HOLD

Begin in the movement starting position and **raise your body so that you are in the sucking-in (internal) position**. Your belly button sucks in and your head and shoulders remain off the floor. Keep your knees tucked into your stomach with your feet off the ground. Your lower back should remain in contact with the floor.

SQUEEZING (EXTERNAL)

SUCKING IN (INTERNAL)

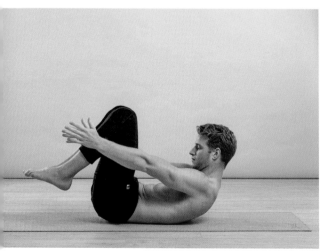

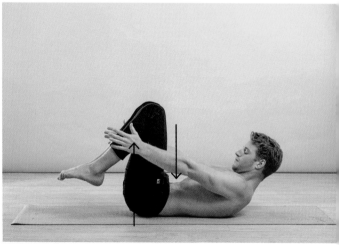

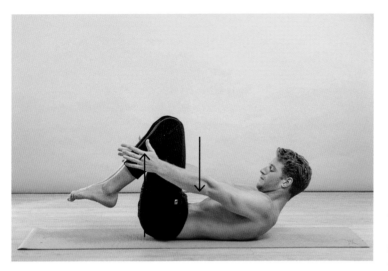

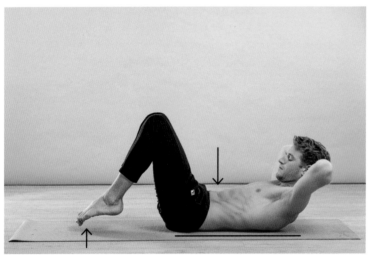

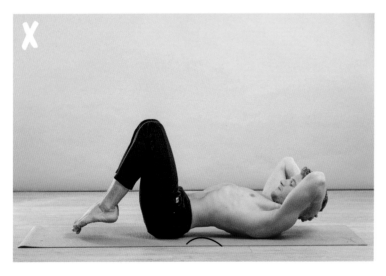

3. ADVANCED STOMACH CONTROL

For Exercise 3, the only change from the previous exercise is that your knees move away from your abdominals and your feet are lowered closer to the floor. You're training yourself to be able to hold the weight of your legs with your stomach muscles. Support your head with your hands (don't push).

1-MINUTE MOVEMENT

Lie on your back on a mat or soft surface with your knees bent and tucking in towards your chest. Place your hands behind your head. **Raise your feet to hover above the floor and raise your head, neck and shoulders. Move between a tuck (squeezing the abdominals) and an advanced-tuck (bringing your hands behind your head and lowering your toes closer to the floor) position**, keeping your feet off the floor and your lower back in contact with the floor throughout.

REMEMBER: Internal means you are sucking your belly button down to the floor; external means you are squeezing your abdominals.

1-MINUTE HOLD

Position yourself in the starting position for the movement and **adopt the internal position**: belly button sucked in, head and shoulders off the floor, feet hovering off the floor, lower back in contact with the floor at all times. Hold.

4. OVERHEAD RIB CONTROL

In Exercise 4, you're going to practise moving your ribs. Grab a mat and a block (or this book) and lie on the ground in your tucked Hollow Body position.

First, I want you to test your spine and shoulder mobility by seeing if you can touch the floor behind you with a block. Initially, it doesn't matter if you don't touch the floor, but eventually you need to be able to get the block to the floor without raising your rib cage from the mat – if your rib cage raises, you've gone too far.

1-MINUTE MOVEMENT
Lying in the tucked Hollow Tuck position (see page 59), **take a block (or book) as high overhead as possible towards the floor behind you.** Your lower back should not leave the floor. **Move your arms forward and back for the full minute.**

1-MINUTE HOLD
Starting in the tucked Hollow Tuck position, pull your ribs closed and suck in your stomach. **Bring your arms overhead, with your ribs sucked in, as far as you can go. Hold.**

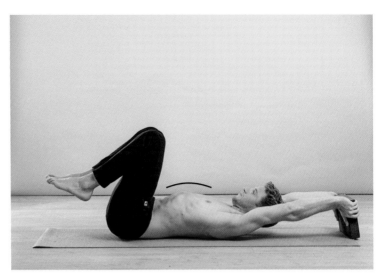

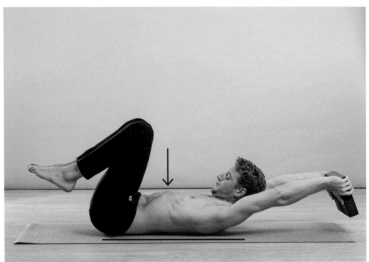

5. PUSH/PULL

For years I attended yoga classes and I wish that somebody had pulled me aside to show me how to do this strength exercise correctly. It wasn't until I came across gymnastics that I could really excel at it.

At first glance you may look at the image and go, "I know this one." Trust me. This is *not* Child's Pose nor the shoulder stretch you're thinking of, although it does look familiar. This is a tough exercise that needs strength and flexibility. There are two things you need to know:

» **PULL** is your stomach sucking in (internal, like in Exercise 1)
» **PUSH** is arms externally rotating (opening) and actively pushing away

IMPORTANT: Do not press your chest down to the floor and collapse into your shoulders – your back must remain flat. You will end up doing more harm than good.

1-MINUTE MOVEMENT

Kneel on all fours on a mat. Extend your arms in front of you, resting on the outsides of your hands, thumbs pointing upwards – this encourages your shoulders to externally rotate (open). **Actively push away with your fingertips (thumbs upwards) and pull in your stomach.** Your chest will lower towards the floor. Don't bend your arms; keep your elbows locked and let the push/pull do the work.

1-MINUTE HOLD

Beginning in the final movement position, **look at your hands and hold, actively pushing away and sucking in your stomach.** As you pull in your stomach, your butt should be directly above the knees. The images below right show what your shoulders should and shouldn't be doing from another angle, in a seated position. In the top photo, the shoulders are rotating in (closing); in the bottom photo, they are rotating out (opening).

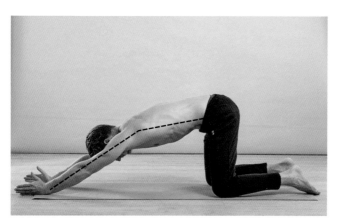

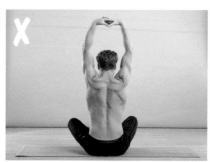

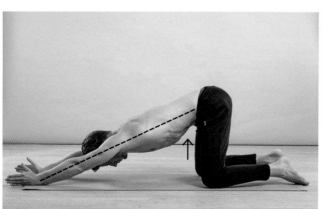

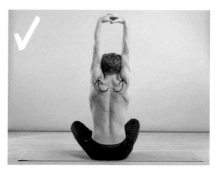

6. LOCKED-LEG PYRAMID

The Locked-leg Pyramid will improve your overhead range – you'll need this in order to perform the Full Hollow Body. I recommend that you get confident with Exercise 5 before doing this exercise, as it's exactly the same thing but with locked legs. If you've ever done yoga, this may look a little like a Downward Dog. It has similarities, but your attention should focus on your shoulders, rather than aiming to get your heels flat on the floor.

In order to practise this exercise properly and safely, you'll need to:
» **PUSH** with your hands
» **PULL** with your stomach

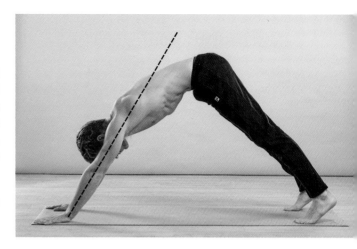

1-MINUTE MOVEMENT
Begin on all fours, hands shoulder-width apart, fingers pointing forwards. **Lift your knees from the ground and come up on your toes, raising your body into the air. From here, press the ground away while sucking in your stomach.** This pushes your butt as high as it will go, lowers your heels and creates a straight line from wrists to butt. Lock your legs to create the pyramid shape. Do all this slowly over the full minute.

1-MINUTE HOLD
Hold your body in the Pyramid you created at the end of the movement, while pushing through the floor and sucking in your stomach. This will flatten your spine and externally rotate your shoulders. Your legs should remain locked throughout.

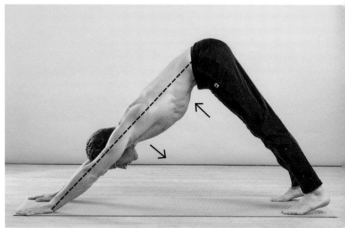

7. SINGLE-LEG HOLLOW BODY

In Exercise 7, you're going to take a look at what your legs are doing when they go straight. Pointing your toes will really help you to squeeze your butt, which is essential in the exercise. Continuing to focus on sucking in your stomach will no longer help you in this exercise – we've got to get the butt involved for you to successfully achieve this progression.

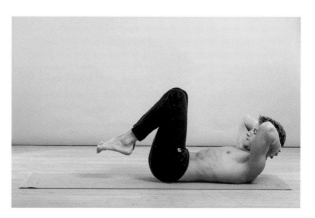

1-MINUTE MOVEMENT

Lie down in the Hollow Tuck (see page 59), suck in your stomach and slightly raise your shoulders from the floor. Place your hands behind your neck (support, don't push). **Extend one leg, point your toes and squeeze your butt, while at the same time lock your leg.** Your extended foot stays slightly off the ground – you should be actively pressing it away from you.

NOTE: It's your tucked leg's job to help keep your stomach sucked in.

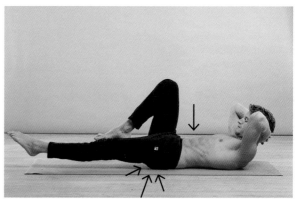

Now, **bring your extended leg back into the tuck position, while at the same time extending the other leg, toes pointed, hovering above the ground**. When that leg is fully extended, slowly bring it back, extending the other leg again. Keep moving each leg slowly alternating legs.

1-MINUTE HOLD

Hold your body in the one-legged position for 30 seconds, then change legs (or spend longer on the side where you feel weaker, if you prefer). Focus on the following:

» Stomach sucked in
» Butt muscles squeezed
» Knees locked
» Toes pointed
» Extended leg locked out

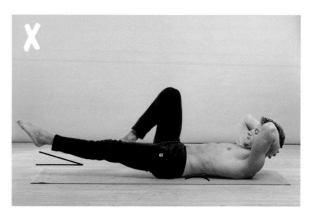

PROGRESSION: Once you are comfortable keeping this hold for 30 seconds on each side, aim for 1 minute on each side instead.

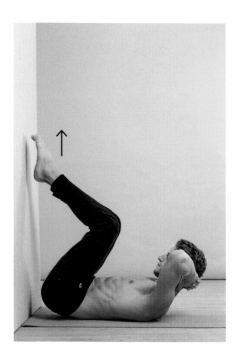

8. THE HOLLOW WALL

The Hollow Wall is designed to test your core strength and leg flexibility at the same time, because each one affects the other.

1-MINUTE MOVEMENT

Start in a Hollow Tuck (see Exercise 2, page 59) with your butt as close to the wall as possible, hands supporting your head. Your aim is to **move from a tuck position into a locked-leg position by extending your legs**. Your feet must not touch the wall and your spine must always remain in contact with the ground. Use the full minute.

1-MINUTE HOLD

Suck in your stomach as much as you can to pull your legs away from the wall. Your spine should remain in contact with the floor and your legs should remain locked and straight. Hold.

TIP: If it seems impossible to keep your feet from dropping against the wall, scooch backwards a little, until you can hold the position comfortably for 1 minute with your back on the floor throughout.

PROGRESSION: When you're ready, move closer to the wall so that your legs rest on the wall in the start position. Then, move them away from the wall and hold for 1 minute.

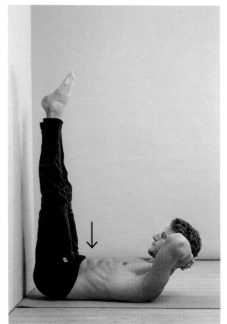

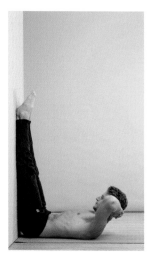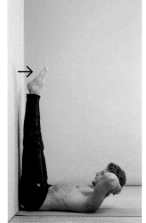

PROGRESSION

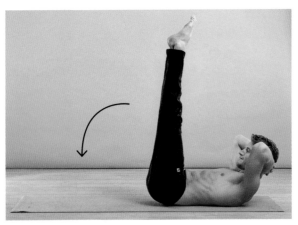

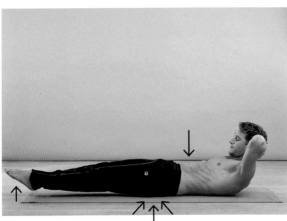

9. DOUBLE-LEG HOLLOW BODY

In Exercise 9, you're going to take a look again at the role of the legs in achieving the Hollow Body. Before you attempt this, make sure you're comfortable with the Single-leg Hollow Body (Exercise 7, page 64).

IMPORTANT: The biggest mistake I see people make during this exercise is to let the rib cage open (see page 61), which puts pressure on your lower back.

1-MINUTE MOVEMENT

Begin with your legs pointing upwards and angled slightly towards your head (as if away from an imaginary wall). From this position, slowly, maintaining a flat back throughout, **lower both your legs simultaneously to the floor, but without letting them touch the floor**. Make sure your lower back is in contact with the floor at all times. Keep moving your legs up and down for the full minute. Don't forget: it's essential to squeeze your butt and suck in your stomach.

TIP: You'll only be able to squeeze your butt once your legs are low to the ground – just make sure you do it at the bottom before bringing your legs back up.

1-MINUTE HOLD

Follow the instructions for the movement, lowering your legs towards the floor. **Keep them slightly off the floor, toes pointed, and hold for as long as you can**, but ideally the whole minute. If you feel you're losing your position and your lower back is arching from the ground, regress to single legs or even tucking the knees in. Focus on keeping:
» Stomach sucked in
» Butt squeezed
» Legs locked
» Toes pointed
» Lower back on the ground

TIP: Place your hands behind your neck to help alleviate any neck tension while you move.

10. BRINGING IT ALL TOGETHER – THE FULL HOLLOW BODY

Exercise 10 will test your shoulder mobility together with your core strength to create the Full Hollow Body. Pulling in your belly button to keep your lower back on the ground will test the core, and taking your arms overhead will determine your shoulder mobility. The aim is to get your arms down to the floor behind you, while your legs are lifted and your back remains in contact with the floor. (As you can see, I was a little restricted in this movement when the photo was taken!)

You may want to start by trying this exercise in a tuck and single-leg position before moving to the Full Hollow. Your priority is to protect your lower back.

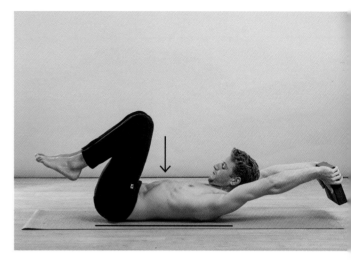

1-MINUTE MOVEMENT

Lie down in the final position for Exercise 4 (see page 61), but with your arms by your sides. **Take your arms as far overhead as you can so that your shoulders externally rotate**. Don't just open your shoulders, but actively press your hands away from you. Holding a block can help. As you press back, your arms will lock and your elbow pits (the insides of your elbows) will face each other. Straighten your legs as you did in the final position for Exercise 9 (opposite). **Move your knees from tucked to straight with arms reaching overhead, keeping your stomach sucked in and your feet off the ground**. Repeat.

1-MINUTE HOLD

Lie down in the fully extended position you achieved in the movement, with your legs hovering above the floor and your arms fully extended and locked behind you – this is the Full Hollow Body. Hold the position for the full minute.

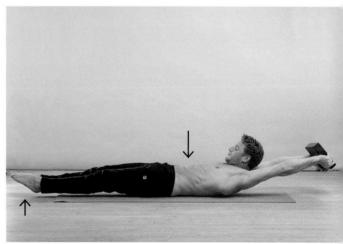

LIFE HACK

OFFICE STRETCH

Take advantage of this life hack while sitting on your office chair. Put your arms behind you and clasp your hands together around the back of your chair. Make sure your:

» Shoulders are stretched back

» Arms are locked

» Belly button is sucked in

This will help to keep your ribs down, just as they are in the Hollow Body. When you first stretch your shoulders back, your rib cage opens. Sucking in your belly button will add more tension to the stretch.

For more advice on how to do this, see www.roger.coach.

FOOD FOR THOUGHT

I remember first being introduced to the Hollow Body several years ago. I was surprised how challenging I found it to keep my lower back on the floor, sucking my stomach in, even in a tuck position.

Before I started training using my own bodyweight for resistance, like most young guys I went to the gym and lifted weights, doing the usual bench-press and biceps-curl exercises that you would expect. I believed this had made me quite strong. However, the Hollow Body revealed what I had actually achieved: I'd become extremely tight and compromised on the natural movement I was born with.

Although my gym background was not a complete waste of time, getting my movement back meant that I needed to spend a lot of time undoing all the physiological changes I'd been through as a result of weight-training and not moving properly.

Like you, I was born with a full range of motion. Knowing that keeps me on track to spend the rest of my life getting that entire range of motion back. People ask me about "becoming" flexible. I simply reply: "You were born flexible; you have just got to invest some time into getting your flexibility back."

I'd never experienced what it was like to suck in my stomach. Sure, I'd done crunches, Planks, even played around with an ab wheel and yoga ball, but I was always bracing my stomach (squeezing my abdominals), not sucking them in the way I talk about doing so for exercise, from the rib cage. Sucking in the stomach is one of the key components for training your body to be super-strong from the inside out.

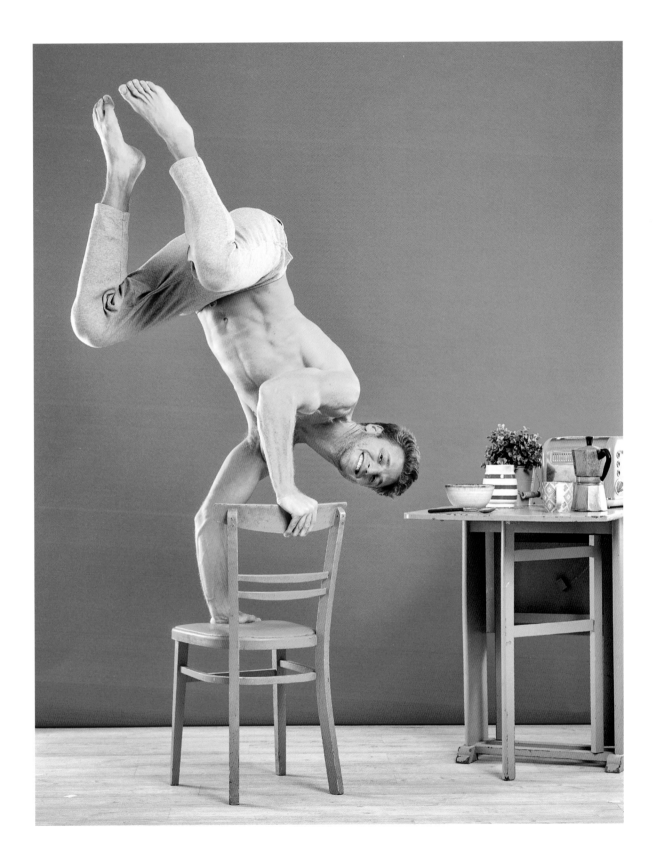

FROG STAND

4

The Frog Stand requires skill. It's important to know right from the off, though, that like the Headstand (see page 112), the Frog Stand is not a balance exercise. It's an exercise that requires you to fail regularly until you are able to do it. When I say fail, I mean fail to understand how it works – but, after some solid practice and correcting yourself as you go, you will have a "Eureka!" moment and everything will click into place.

The Frog Stand is about building your house on a solid foundation. Simply trying to balance over and over again will not only cause you to potentially injure yourself, but you'll lack the ability to progress any further (which you'll want to do if you want to get to achieve a Headstand or the move on the cover of this book, see Take Off, page 124). It's a case of taking your time; building up, progression by progression and piece by piece. You've spent most of your life on your feet, so – be patient: it may take a while to get used to having the weight on your hands.

I love this exercise because as well as requiring me to be fully conscious, it also helps me to regain some confidence in my ability to move out of my comfort zone. Plus it has the physical benefits of making me stronger, and of training new neural pathways in my body.

How often do you stand there and wonder, "How am I able to stand?" You don't. I promise you that it took you months of consistent, daily hard work to stand without thinking about it. Treat this exercise like your toddler self did when you wanted to be able to stand up. Practise, practise, practise and one day you'll master it forever.

BENEFITS
- » Improved wrist mobility
- » Increased arm, back and shoulder strength
- » Core strength
- » Increased confidence
- » Better awareness of your body

HOW TO MOVE
Choose 5 exercises from this book for your 10-minutes-a-day training. Identify the exercise in this section that you need to improve and repeat until you are able to progress to the next exercise. One exercise comprises both a 1-minute slow movement and a 1-minute static hold.

FOOD FOR THOUGHT
An established neural pathway is the reason why right-handed people can't initially write with their left hand and vice versa. People achieve ambidexterity by training themselves to write with their opposite hand. With a new movement or balance, you're not necessarily training specific muscles you're moving repetitively to rewire your brain and create new neural pathways in order to embed the movement in your ability and become a master at it. Just like standing.

1. HAND POWER

Want to wake up tomorrow with neck ache? Nope, nor do I. So let's get the hand positioning right. If your hands are not supporting you fully, then your head will do the work instead – and that means neck ache. If throughout any of these first exercises you experience neck pain, it's a sign you're not following the progressions in the right order.

1-MINUTE MOVEMENT

Start by grabbing yourself a soft mat or two. Position the mats one on top of the other (if necessary), with the stacked short ends against a wall. Kneel up facing the wall. The first shape that you want to create is this: **your head and neck are inverted right up against the wall; your hands are pressed into the floor either side of your knees; your elbows are bent into right angles and pulled in by your sides**. The aim is to **raise one knee at a time and place it on the equivalent elbow**. Switch over, raising the other knee, and continue for the full minute.

1-MINUTE HOLD

Adopt the start position for the movement. Then, **raise one knee and hold it on the equivalent elbow for 30 seconds**. Lower it to the ground and repeat with the other knee and elbow. If you're feeling a little more advanced, challenge yourself to do 1 minute on each side.

When you come out of the hold, ask yourself: do I feel tension in my neck or head? If the answer is yes, then you need to train your hands and arms to take more of the support. Your head, although a point of contact with the floor, is not a main support for your body.

IMPORTANT: Remember that the aim of this support exercise is to teach you hand positioning. The knuckle of your index finger presses into the floor, giving you enough power to support your knees on your elbows. In addition, make sure you keep your elbows pressed into your sides (see below, right photos).

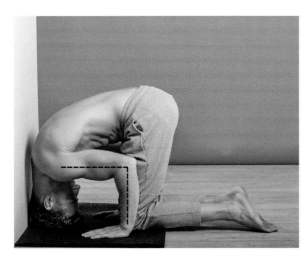

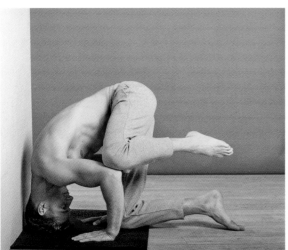

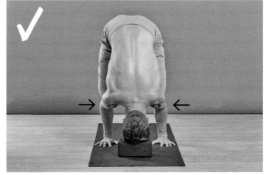

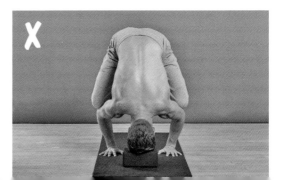

2. ARM POWER WITH STRAIGHT LEGS

In Exercise 2, you're going to press your legs straight while keeping you arms, head and elbows in the same place: head against the wall, elbows raised and by your sides, forearms at right angles to the floor. It can help to tiptoe your feet forwards so that your upper back can rest on the wall. However, if this causes pressure on your head, walk your feet back a bit.

IMPORTANT: Your head should be right up against the wall – don't bring it away from the wall, as this will cause you to roll on your neck.

1-MINUTE MOVEMENT
Kneel facing the wall, invert your head and neck up against the wall, press your hands into the floor either side of your knees and bend your elbows. **Slowly straighten your legs, pushing into the floor with your hands, raising your knees and keeping the tops of your toes on the ground**. Keep your forearms at right angles to the floor. Raise and lower for the full minute. Don't let your elbows fall out to the sides.

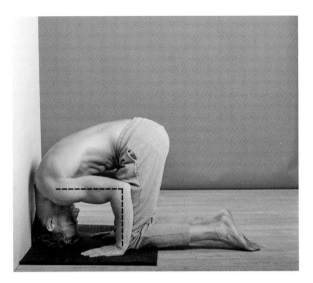

1-MINUTE HOLD
Adopt the starting position for the movement, then **raise your knees and hold your body in the straight-leg position**. If this is too much for you at first, bend your knees slightly. Your leg flexibility and core strength will have an impact on this exercise. Go through the following points while you are performing the hold:
» Head tight up against the wall
» Forearms at right angles to the ground
» Elbows pulled into the body
» Hands firmly pressed into the floor
» Belly button sucked in
» Upper back rested on the wall

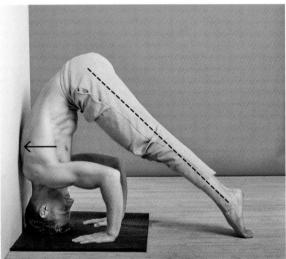

3. KNEE TO ELBOW

In Exercise 3, you're going to position one knee on top of one elbow from a straight-leg position. Some people experience pain in their wrists, which is the body compensating until your arms are strong enough to hold the position. Taking your hands slightly closer to the wall should help. The goal is *not* to push through pain, but to learn about your body through the sensations you feel.

Your starting positions are the same as in exercises 1 and 2: your head should be up against the wall, your wrists beside your knees and your hands pressed firmly into the floor.

1-MINUTE MOVEMENT
From the starting position, raise your knees so that your legs are straight. **Bend one knee and place it on the equivalent elbow, then lower it back into the straight position.** Repeat using the other leg. Keep alternating legs for the full minute.

REMEMBER: Press firmly through your hands to keep the pressure off your head. Your arms should feel some fatigue after this exercise.

1-MINUTE HOLD
Adopt the starting position for the movement, with the legs straight. **In turn, hold each knee for 30 seconds on the equivalent elbow.** For more advanced progression, try holding for 1 minute on each side.

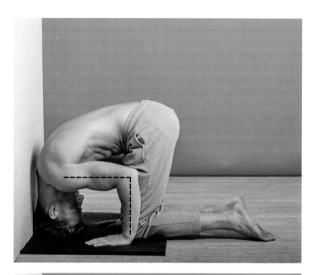

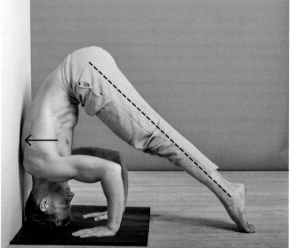

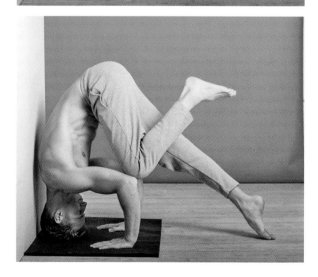

4. BENT-ARM LEAN

In Exercise 4, you're going to come away from the wall and attempt a position that directly relates to the Frog Stand, helping to build the strength in your arms and teaching you the recognise the position of your forearms.

1-MINUTE MOVEMENT

Kneel on a mat, then put your hands on the floor, shoulders directly above your wrists. **Bend your elbows, leaning forwards with your upper body so that it lowers towards the floor.** Stop when your forearms and upper arms form a right angle at your elbow. Your nose and chest should be off the floor. Keep your elbows pulled in – this is crucial for a solid base. Move slowly up and down between straight and bent arms. Your knees remain on the floor throughout.

1-MINUTE HOLD

Starting on all fours with your arms straight, **lean forwards and lower down into the bent-arm position, so that your upper arms and forearms form a right angle. Hold**. Your elbows should be pulled in and your forearms directly over your wrists.

FOOD FOR THOUGHT

I used to do push-ups when I was younger. Then, I learned that my very bad habits made it impossible to transfer to a correct Frog Stand. It took me longer to relearn an elbows-in push-up than if I'd never done push-ups in the first place. Training with impeccable technique and getting the basics in place not only prevents injury, but ensures quick progress. In this book, each exercise leads on to the next one, building up your progress to the ultimate exercise in the sequence. In the Frog Stand, understanding the lean is fundamental to success. And bonus! It will also help you with Headstand and the L-Sits (see pages 112 and 128). As my uncle used to say, "Stuff leads to stuff."

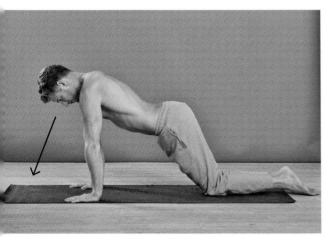

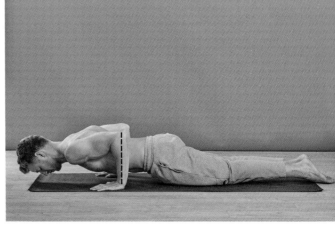

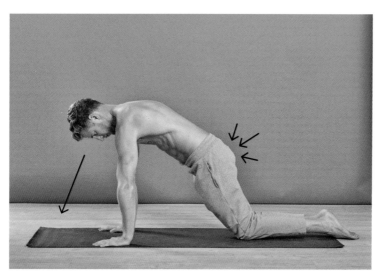

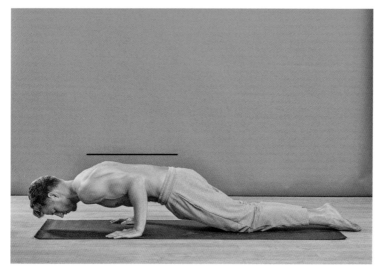

5. BENT-ARM LEAN WITH TUCKED PELVIS

For Exercise 5, you're going to repeat Exercise 4 (see page 75), only this time you're going to tuck in your pelvis fully (see page 54).

1-MINUTE MOVEMENT

Start on all fours on a mat, pelvis tucked in, butt squeezed. **Bend your arms at the elbows and lean forwards, keeping your pelvis tucked, lowering towards the floor**, just as you did in Exercise 4 (see page 75). Pause for a few seconds in the bent-arm position, holding the right angle at your elbow. Your elbows should be pulled in close to your body and your forearms directly over your wrists. Move slowly up and down between bent arm and straight arm, keeping your pelvis tucked.

REMEMBER: Keeping your elbows pulled in and leaning forwards with your body is crucial for creating a solid base for the Frog Stand.

1-MINUTE HOLD

Start on your knees in a tucked-pelvis and straight-arm position, then **lean forwards and lower down into the bent-arm position** so that each arm creates a right angle at the elbow. Hold.

6. BENT-ARM LEAN WITH STRAIGHT LEG

In Exercise 6, you're going to lower into a position that directly matches the Frog Stand, but this time you're going to start in a regular Plank but with an untucked pelvis. These positions form what are essentially Front Support push-ups.

1-MINUTE MOVEMENT

Starting in a Plank position with an untucked pelvis (see page 55), **lower yourself to the floor and pause with your arms bent, creating a right angle at the elbow**. Move slowly up and down, leaning forwards as you lower. Only your toes and hands are in contact with the floor.

1-MINUTE HOLD

Begin in the start position for the movement and **lower yourself to the floor, until your arms form right angles and only your toes and hands are in contact with the floor. Hold**. Your elbows should be pulled in close to your body and your forearms should be directly over your wrists.

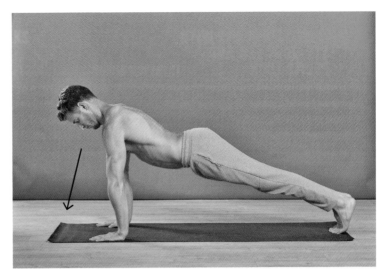

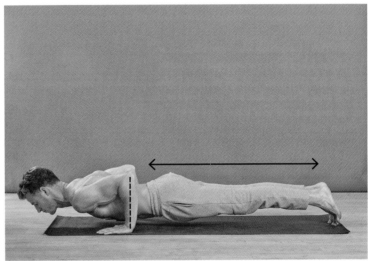

9. ROLLING ONTO A SINGLE BLOCK

Before you begin Exercise 9, make sure you're confident with Exercise 8: you're going to perform it again, but with only one block (or fewer blocks if you had more than two last time). Reducing the number of blocks will increase the amount you need to roll forwards before your head touches the floor. This is a good exercise to practise for the sake of confidence and getting the right technique.

1-MINUTE MOVEMENT
Starting in a tiptoe squat as in Exercise 8 (see page 79), **place your knees just above your elbows, bend your elbows and roll forwards until your head touches the block.**

1-MINUTE HOLD
From the tiptoe squat starting position, **roll forwards to place your head on the block**. Your knees should be on your elbows, forehead on the block and feet off the ground. Hold for the full minute.

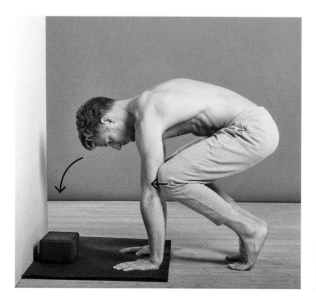

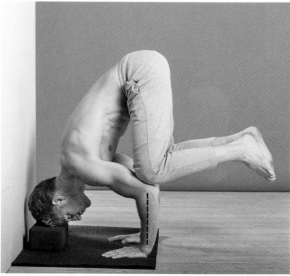

10. FROG STAND

This is it – the full Frog Stand. Don't forget that there's nothing wrong with failing ungracefully. I took a good few months and I learned to become really good at failing. If your Frog Stands are looking something like the image on the right, I'm pleased to tell you that you're on the right track.

1-MINUTE MOVEMENT

Starting in a tiptoe squat, **place your knees on top of your elbows and lean forwards**. This time, there's no block, so just keep going, slowly, until you find the position as if you're block were there. Focus on the following:
» Hands pressed into the floor
» Elbows squeezed in
» Heels squeezed to butt
Go forward and back like this for the full minute.

1-MINUTE HOLD

The more you practise the roll movement, the more you need to slow it down – until eventually you **stop altogether, coming into a hold that is the Frog Stand**. Your butt is in the air, your elbows are above wrists and your feet are pointing behind you, with your knees resting on your elbows.

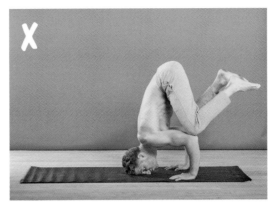

GETTING IT WRONG IS GOOD

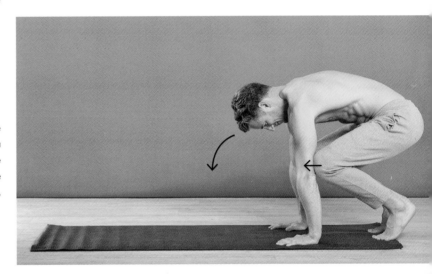

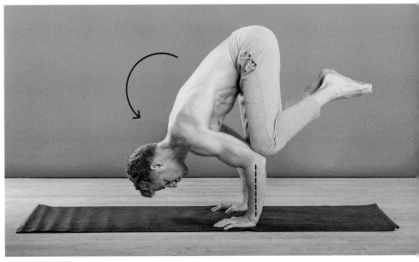

LIFE HACK

ROLLING AROUND

Do the words roly poly spring to mind? Well, if you Google the term "roly poly", apparently it's so outdated you get an image of a cartoon bug. I think I remember doing it at school, although I didn't really have a clue what I was doing. So, your life hack is to roll on the floor. Really, that's it: roll on the floor in as many ways as you can. When you've had enough of that, you can try a Frog-stand Roll (if you like).

Find yourself a nice soft surface and some clothes you don't mind messing up a bit and play around like a toddler. Training doesn't have to be a structured process – it can also be about being comfortable and creating movements as you go. You'll always shy away from the Frog Stand unless you aren't afraid to fall over. You might say, "Roger, but what if I injure myself?" Well, this is my response...

FROG-STAND ROLLS

Frog-stand Rolls are a test of strength, technique and confidence. If you've moved slowly and carefully through all the progressions to Frog Stand, this exercise will make perfect sense. When your knees are on top of your elbows and your elbows are pulled into the sides of your body, you create a gap. This gap is where your head is going to go for the roll.

TIP: Make sure you have a soft surface for practising this exercise. Remember – multiple failures are the path to success!

During the roll, your head never touches the floor. Never! If it does, your elbows have collapsed. You cannot roll with collapsed elbows, because then you have nothing supporting you. Just like

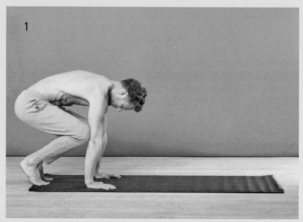

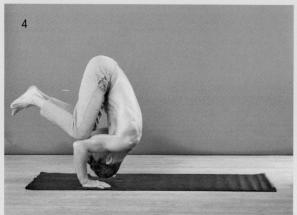

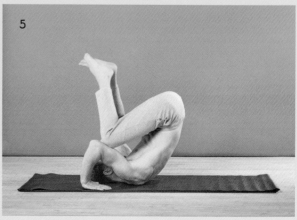

with a Headstand (see page 112), your hands pressing firmly into the floor and your elbows pulling in is what supports you.

So, starting in a tiptoe squat (see page 79), place your knees on top of your elbows, lean forwards and roll through, putting your head through the gap in your arms. As you roll, squeeze your chin into your chest, press your hands to the floor and squeeze your elbows into your body. Over and through.

FOOD FOR THOUGHT

Every time you choose to sit down for any long period of time, you're harming yourself. You will become increasingly stiff and inflexible, and speed up the process of growing old and fragile. Instead, like a toddler, roll about without a care. If you progress to Frog-stand Rolls, you'll have the added benefit of conquering any fear of moving into Frog Stand, too.

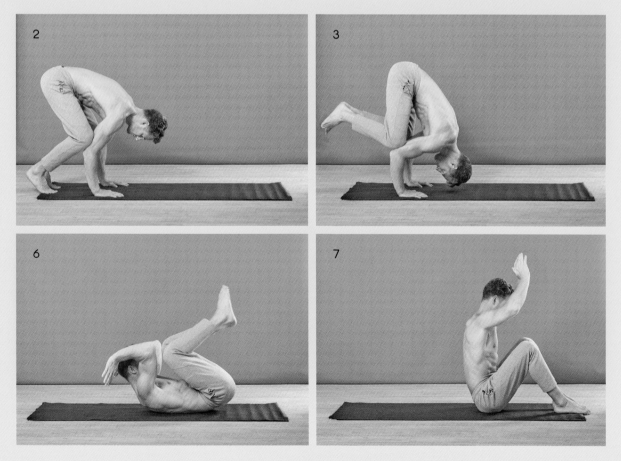

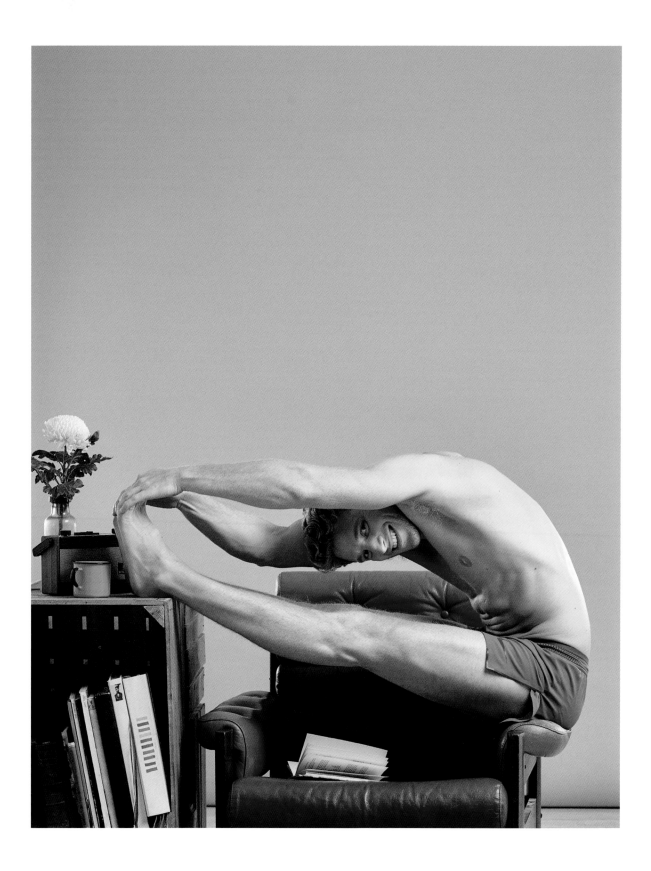

5

LEGS, LEGS, LEGS

We tend to think of flexibility as something that we practise as a warm-up or after a workout, but earlier on in the book we discovered how we were born with full flexibility – a full range of motion – in our joints. Getting that flexibility back and maintaining it is absolutely essential for your body's health all the time.

When I first started exercising, I would say my exercise would be divided between 10-per-cent flexibility and 90-per-cent strength. However, now I promote exercise that is 80-per-cent flexibility and 20-per-cent strength. Why? Because the strength elements become effortless when you a reach a practical level of flexibility.

If you lack flexibility in your body, your chances of injuring yourself are at a higher level when exercising. Tight muscles and joints cause injuries and pull you into postures that not only hurt but leave you feeling depressed. This chapter focuses on getting the motion back in your legs.

BENEFITS
» Improved leg flexibility (obviously)
» Improved spine flexibility
» Improved hip flexibility
» Leaning to cope with uncomfortable feelings
» Improved body awareness

HOW TO MOVE
Choose 5 exercises from this book for your 10-minutes-a-day training. Identify the exercise in this section that you need to improve and repeat until you are able to progress to the next exercise. One exercise comprises both a 1-minute slow movement and a 1-minute static hold.

1. LEG LOCKING

Leg locking is integral to the exercises for leg flexibility. In fact, it is integral to the majority of exercises in the book! Therefore, in Exercise 1, I'm going to show you how to fully lock your legs. If you have a think through all the leg exercises, or even day-to-day activities, you do or have done in the past, you'll probably find that your legs have been bent most of the time: lunges, squats, walking, jogging, running, jumping and so on. No wonder touching your toes while keeping your legs straight has become so challenging. You've trained your legs to become good at bending. That's great – but they need to be good at straight-leg motions, too.

1-MINUTE MOVEMENT

Sit on a mat with your back straight and your legs straight out in front of you, feet flexed. Position your hands behind you, fingers pointing backwards. **Press the backs of your knees into the mat so that the heels of your feet raise off the ground.** Leg locking happens at the point where your heels are suspended above the mat. You are not lifting your legs here, just squeezing the muscles at the front of your legs enough so that your knees press downwards and your heels lift off the mat.

1-MINUTE HOLD

Begin in the same position as for the movement. Then, **squeeze your leg muscles and press the backs of your knees into the mat, keeping your feet flexed, so that both your heels leave the ground. Hold.** You may also want to try this with pointed toes, too.

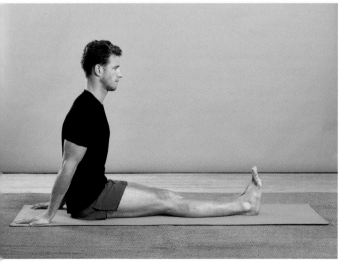

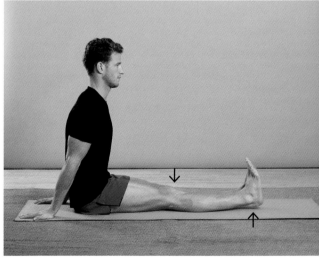

2. FLEXIBILITY TEST 1

In Exercise 2, you're going to use the length of your mat to test your leg flexibility.

Your objective is to get your fingertips to touch the floor while keeping your legs spread wide and locked straight.

IMPORTANT: Stay focused on keeping the fronts of your legs locked even if you have to go further forwards to get your fingertips on the ground.

1-MINUTE MOVEMENT

Lay out your mat with its length perpendicular to your body. Stand with your toes at the edge of the mat, then spread your legs as wide as they will go. Lean forwards, legs locked, until your fingertips touch the floor.

Keeping your fingertips in contact with the floor, **move between a small bend in your knees and locked legs**. Small movements will help you feel the difference between locked and unlocked legs.

1-MINUTE HOLD

Standing in your wide-leg position, **bend forwards and place your fingertips on the mat. Lock your legs and hold.**

REMEMBER: Your fingertips should always remain in contact with the floor.

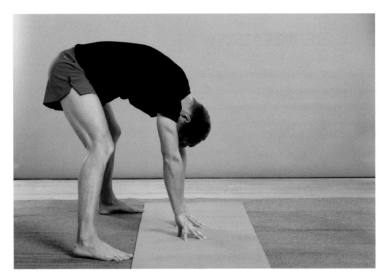

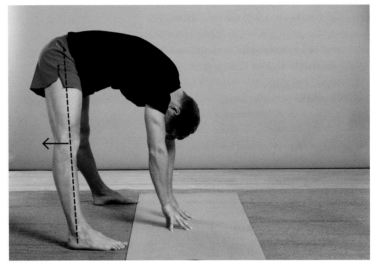

5. NARROW-LEG ROCKS

Like the previous exercise, Exercise 5 requires the same balance of push (from the fingertips) and pull (from pulling in your stomach).

1-MINUTE MOVEMENT

Begin in the starting position for the movement in Exercise 3 (see page 88). **Keeping your legs and arms straight, rock back and forth between the "lean forwards" and the "press back".** When you lean forwards, your shoulders stack above your hands. When you press back, aim to get your butt as far back as possible without letting your fingertips leave the floor.

TIP: As you improve, walk your fingertips closer to your feet and try again.

1-MINUTE HOLD

Stand with your feet as wide as the narrow width of the mat, **lean forwards and press your fingertips into the floor. Pull in your belly button and press your hips as far back as you can without your fingertips leaving the floor. Hold.**

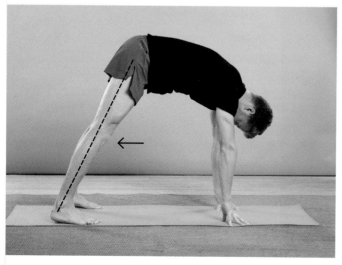
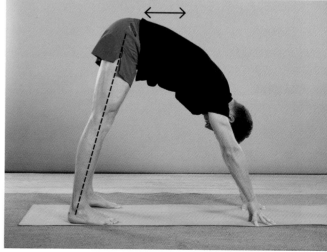

6. ACHILLES HEEL

The Achilles Heel of all exercises. This one should hit a slightly different spot in the back of the legs then you're used to when working with your feet flat on the ground. For this exercise, you'll need a couple of different block sizes or a couple of books to help you get into it.

1-MINUTE MOVEMENT

Start in a standing position. Place the pads of one foot on top of your lower block or book, keeping your heel in contact with the ground, grab the support block you're going to be using and place that on the ground, holding onto the other end of it for support. **Keeping both knees locked, slowly move between a bent arm and a straight arm,** with both feet facing forwards for 30 seconds. Swap sides and repeat using the other leg.

1-MINUTE HOLD

Lower into position keeping the knees locked and hold for 30 seconds. Swap sides and repeat.

NOTE: The lower the support your are holding, the more challenging the exercise will become. Work towards getting your fingertips, then your palms on the ground as you improve.

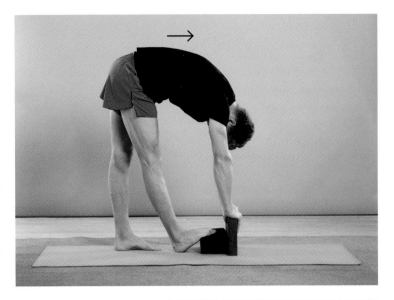

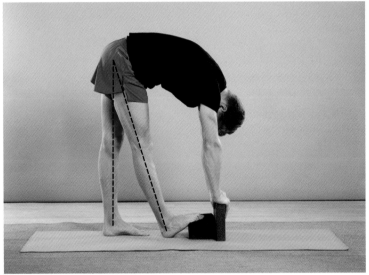

7. SQUAT TO STAND

In Exercise 7, you're going to work into the stretch from a squat position. It's not imperative here that you're able to get all the way down to the squat. You'll find that the more you do this, the better you get at squatting anyway.

At the beginning, move as much as you can up and down through the range of squat to standing while keeping your fingertips in the same place.

1-MINUTE MOVEMENT

With your feet as wide as the narrow width of your mat, drop into the squat position, allowing your chest to rest on your thighs. Place your fingertips on the floor in front of you, far enough forwards that it will allow you to straighten your legs fully. **Keeping your feet and fingertips in position, move slowly upward between the squat and the legs-locked position.**

1-MINUTE HOLD

Begin as for the movement. **Raise up and hold your body in the straight-legged position.** Work on keeping your butt behind your feet.

TIP: If you find these exercises difficult, try resting your fingertips on a block instead of the floor.

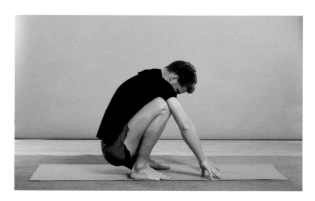

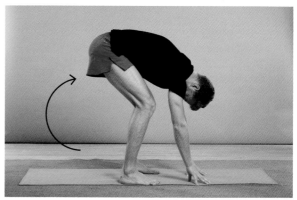

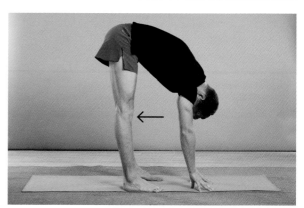

8. ADVANCED SQUAT TO STAND

In Exercise 8, you're going to work into the stretch from a squat position in the same way as in Exercise 7 but this time with your palms on the floor instead of your fingertips.

1-MINUTE MOVEMENT

With your feet as wide as the narrow width of your mat, drop into the squat position, allowing your chest to rest on your thighs. Place your fingertips on the floor in front of you, far enough forwards that it will allow you to straighten your legs fully. **Keeping your feet and fingertips in position, move slowly upward between the squat and the legs-locked position.**

1-MINUTE HOLD

Begin as for the movement. **Raise up and hold your body in the straight-legged position.** Work on keeping your butt behind your feet.

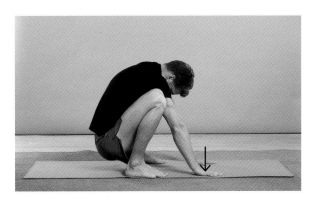

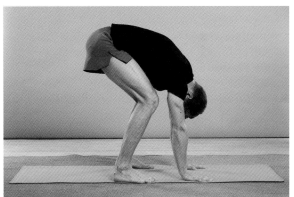

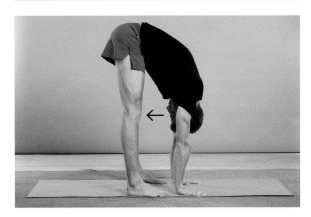

9. PULLING INTO POSITION

In Exercise 9, you'll need a solid or immovable object – something like a radiator firmly attached to a wall, or bedposts – in front of you because you're going to use this to pull into position. Find somewhere you have space to get your legs as wide as possible, too.

1-MINUTE MOVEMENT

Sit facing your solid object, and spread your legs as wide as possible. The aim is to get your upper body as far forwards as you can. **Hold onto your object and pull forwards, bending your elbows and pulling your upper body towards the object**. The movement should feel as though you are pushing your butt backwards into an untucked pelvis (see page 40).

1-MINUTE HOLD

Your goal is to get your chest as far forwards as possible using a straight spine. Try not to fold down. **Press your butt backwards into an untucked pelvis and pull your chest forwards.** Take care not to extend your neck – the movement is in your spine, pelvis and chest. Once you are as far forwards as you can go, hold for the full minute.

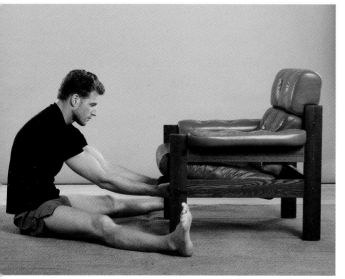

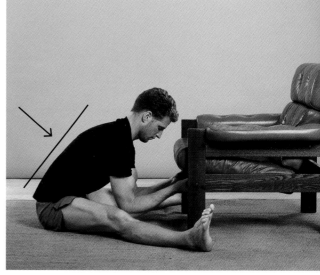

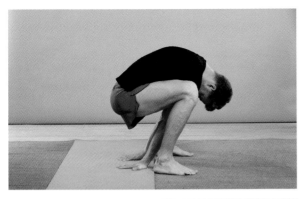

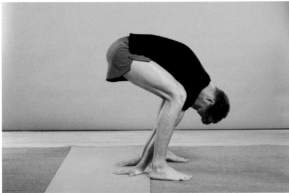

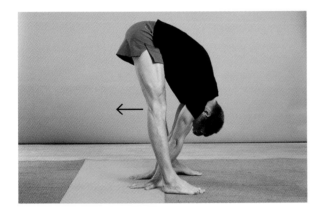

10. BACKWARDS PALMS

You'll find for this exercise that it's easier to work with your legs wider. To get into position, you can bend your knees as much as you need to – the objective is to start to straighten your legs without your palms leaving their start position. The "space" for this exercise comes as a result of sucking in your belly button to straighten your legs.

1-MINUTE MOVEMENT

Stand with your feet as wide as you need to in front of a mat. Bend your knees and place your palms facing backwards on top of the mat. **Move slowly between bent leg and straight leg** while keeping the palms pressed into the mat. You can rock backwards and forwards in this movement, as you did in exercises 4 and 5 (see pages 89 and 90), but your main priority is to lock your legs as you reach the top. Over time, as the movement starts to become more achievable, bring your feet a little closer together. Eventually, you will be able to bring your feet together and still keep your palms on the floor.

1-MINUTE HOLD

Using the movement starting position, find a width for your legs where you can comfortably **keep your palms pressed into the mat and your legs locked. Hold for the full minute**. Bring your feet closer together as you improve.

ADVANCED EXERCISE: When your feet are so close together that you can't comfortably fit your arms through your legs, put your hands either side of your feet.

LIFE HACKS

BEDROCKS

It was a must for me to put a life hack using your bed in the book for three very valid reasons:

» You're likely to have a bed, so it's very accessible
» Your bed is likely to be very comfortable to stretch on
» Whenever and wherever you travel, a bed will be available

Most of us spend between five and nine hours on or in a bed every night, so I'm sure you can find a minute or two each night for improving your flexibility.
For more advice on how to do this, see www.roger.coach.

BED STRETCH

Lie face down on your bed, and open your feet out as wide as possible. Push yourself backwards until you are straddling the bed and you feel a stretch in your thighs. As you advance, you'll be able to push all the way backwards to sitting forwards while keeping your legs straight.

FOOD FOR THOUGHT

There is a theory that when we are unconscious, we are able to do the splits. Now I can't confirm whether there's any truth to this theory, but this is what I take from that statement: the only thing stopping you from stretching further is your nervous system. It's a very clever system that has been put in place to protect you from hurting yourself, especially if you have been injured.

I think that knowing that it is just the nervous system protecting you will help you to relax into stretches. This is why they always say "breathe" in yoga classes – it does help!

Breathing is not the only thing that helps, though. Distracting the mind – watching TV, having a conversation, thinking about what you have to do tomorrow, even counting the leaves on the trees – helps, too. I know this doesn't sound very yoga-like and that's why I'm not teaching you to be a yogi, but the element of distraction can work wonders.

Think of it like this. Your brain can take in only so much information at once. Did you notice the type font on this page, or the kind of paper the book has been printed on, and what about the bird singing outside or how many times you have blinked in the last 60 seconds? I bet you never think about blinking even though you do it all day. I bet you're thinking about blinking now. Weird, isn't it? Now it's hard to get away from thinking about blinking.

For me, when yogis tell us to focus on the breath, they're really encouraging us to use the art of distraction and prioritisation; to distract the mind from prioritising the feeling of the stretch. I know this sounds a bit crazy, but if someone punched you in the face mid-stretch, in a millisecond the pain of the stretch would vanish. Your body focuses on the biggest priority. So, find a new priority away from the uncomfortable. Think about whatever gets you to complete your time – and then give yourself a lovely piece of chocolate cake as a reward afterwards. Mmmmmm, cake. Now, there is food for thought.

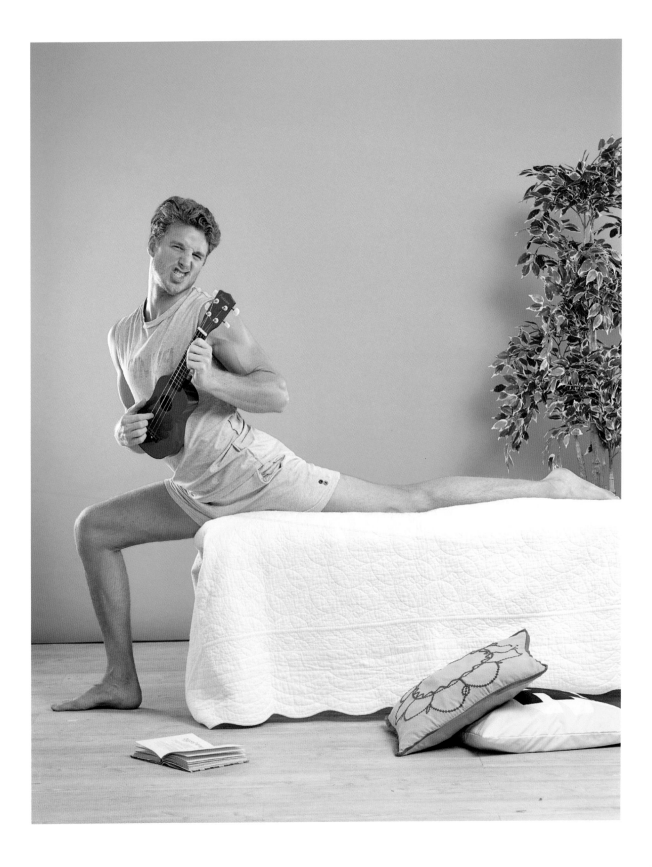

HIP ACTION

Very young children are able to put their big toes in their mouth. It appears to be a basic movement that we're gifted with. When was the last time you tried this, or walked into the gym to see somebody else trying it? You can't remember a time, right? However, it's actually a great test of hip flexibility or, more precisely, "lack of" flexibility. All-round hip flexibility is essential for a healthy body. Tight and weak muscles in the hips can cause all sorts of lower-back and mobility problems, from acute pain to prolonged injury.

What do sprinters, gymnasts and dancers all have in common? I'll tell you. They all have powerful buttocks and flexible hips. So, let's get stuck in and introduce some good exercises that will get your hips moving better again in no time. *Shakira! Shakira!*

BENEFITS
- » The ability to get up from the floor when you're older
- » All-round hip flexibility and mobility
- » Maximising the use of all the joints you have
- » Spine flexibility and mobility
- » Reverses the damage caused by years of sedentary behaviour
- » Improved relationship with uncomfortable feelings
- » Improved body awareness

HOW TO MOVE
Choose 5 exercises from this book for your 10-minutes-a-day training. Identify the exercise in this section that you need to improve and repeat until you are able to progress to the next exercise. One exercise comprises both a 1-minute slow movement and a 1-minute static hold.

FOOD FOR THOUGHT
Before you get stuck into some Hip Action, I'd like to mention a rather important point that I believe is missing from most exercise books.

You're more than likely to have this question pop up in your mind at some point: "Am I stretching correctly?" There is a very simple answer to this. "If you feel a stretch, you are stretching." You might also ask: "Roger, where should I be feeling this?" My reply is always the same. "Where do you feel it?" In other words, there is no "should". We are not all the same. I can guarantee there are some exercises in this book where you don't feel any stretch or you have to move in a slightly different way to get the same stretch.

Do all your friends love the same sports, movies or foods that you do? We all have different tastes and we all have different feelings about things. The question on your mind should be, "Where have I become tight? What stretches work best for me?" You are unique.

1. CROSS-LEGGED SIT

People sitting crossed-legged on the floor is one of the first things you'll notice if you've ever walked into a yoga class. Or a pre-school class.

It's one of those positions that is very natural to us. I have met people who work full-time desk jobs, never do yoga or stretch themselves and sit like this extremely comfortably. However, if you've stopped sitting like it for some time, returning to it can be very challenging. Several years ago, in my first yoga class, my knees were so high they were nearly touching my ears and they really hurt (not in a nice way). It was compensation.

A great way to get around this pain issue is to increase the distance between your feet and your hips, or to raise your hips off the ground by sitting on a block or a book. Whichever option you choose, sitting with knee pain will *not* improve over time. Sit to feel a stretch, not pain.

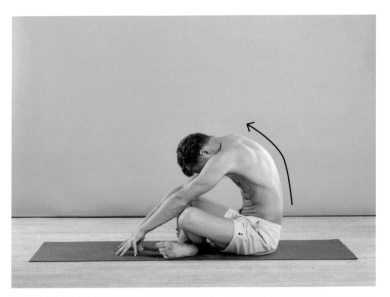

1-MINUTE MOVEMENT

Sit in a pain-free crossed-legged position, with your fingertips on the floor in front of you. If it feels more comfortable, put your fingertips or palms on a block instead. From this position, **move your body between a flexed (rounded) spine and an extended (straight) spine for 30 seconds before alternately crossing your legs.** Your butt should remain in contact with the floor or this will not be challenging; and your arms should remain straight. If you feel any knee pain, slide your butt further back, away from your feet to allow your front leg to come square with the floor.

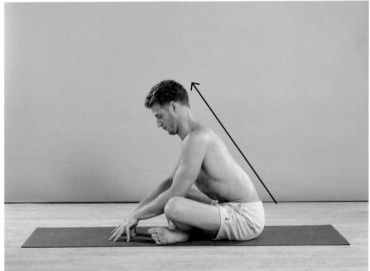

TIP: You can move your hands forwards to make this exercise more challenging.

1-MINUTE HOLD

Hold your body in the extended spine position for 30 seconds on each leg. Focus on:

» Butt on the floor
» Back flat
» Hands remain on the floor
» Front leg square to the floor

2. SIDE BODY STRETCH

For Exercise 2, you're going to use the crossed-legged position to stretch the side of your body. I place my elbows on the floor. You may prefer to position them in your lap if that gives you the best stretch in the side of your body. Keep your butt on the floor throughout.

1-MINUTE MOVEMENT

Sit cross-legged. Place one elbow down in your preferred position. Place your other hand on the equivalent knee, elbow relaxed. **Straighten that elbow so that you move slowly between a bent arm and straight arm**. Move from one side to the other and swap legs, too. Aim for 30 seconds on each side, but if you feel tighter on one side than the other, give that side more time.

1-MINUTE HOLD

Sit crossed-legged and adopt the starting position for the movement. **Press down on your knee to straighten your arm, and hold**. If at first the stretch is quite intense, do 20 seconds each side, working your way up to a full 30 seconds each side as you improve.

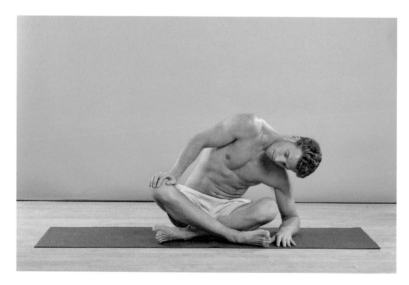

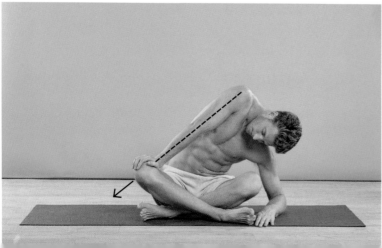

3. THREADED FOLDING STRETCH

For Exercise 3, you're going to thread your elbows under your knees with the soles of your feet together. You may not be able to get your elbows to touch the floor at first, so just go to wherever you can until you feel a stretch. On the other hand, you may not feel any stretch at all – in which case, reposition yourself until you find it.

REMEMBER: Don't ask the question, "Where should I feel this?" There is no general answer. Ask yourself, "Where *do* I feel this?" and then adjust accordingly.

1-MINUTE MOVEMENT
Sit upright on a mat with your legs out in front of you. Bring the soles of your feet together, bending your knees and allowing them to fall to the side. Bend forwards and thread your arms under your knees to hold your feet. **Fold forwards, bringing your forehead towards your feet**. Move slowly between sitting up tall and folding forwards for 1 minute.

1-MINUTE HOLD
From the movement starting position, thread your arms through your legs to grab your feet. **Fold forwards as much as you can until you find a stretch that has the right intensity for you. Hold.**

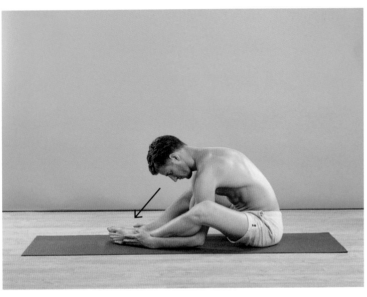

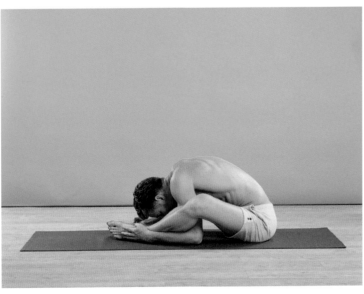

4. SIDE TWIST – SHOULDER TO FLOOR

For exercises 4 and 5, you're going to attempt two different versions of twisting stretches.

What you're doing here is a twist that doesn't move the square line of your body, but results in a stretch in the outside of your hips. It's possible that when you come out of the twist, you'll feel you've stretched your upper body (perhaps your upper back), too.

1-MINUTE MOVEMENT

Lie on your back on a mat, knees bent, feet on the floor and arms by your sides. Put the foot of your right leg on your left knee, then allow both knees to fall to your left so that the left leg is on the floor. Hold your right foot with your left hand. Straighten your right arm and sweep and extend it upwards along the floor. Turn to face your right hand. Roll into the twist, keeping the underneath of the shoulder of your straightened arm on the floor. **Slowly sweep your extended arm up and down, working into the area where you feel the most stretch.** Your goal is to get your arm as high as you can on the upwards sweep. It doesn't matter if the knee of your bent leg raises slightly from the floor. Swap sides during the minute, spending the most time on the side that feels tighter.

1-MINUTE HOLD

Adopt the starting position for the movement, with your straight arm extended as far as it will go. You need to keep your hip off the ground for the stretch to be at its most effective. Practise on both sides, spending the most time on the side that feels tighter.

REMEMBER: Your priority is to keep the shoulder of your extended arm on the floor throughout.

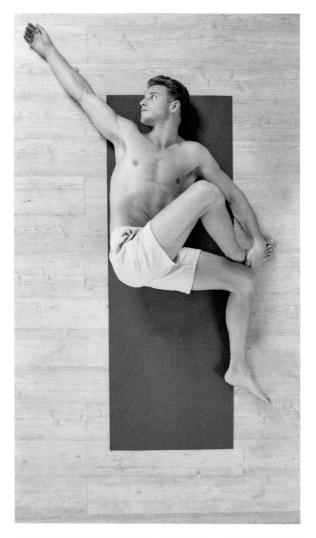

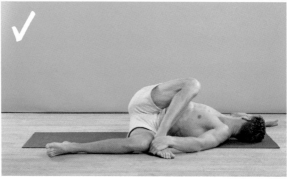

FROM ANOTHER ANGLE

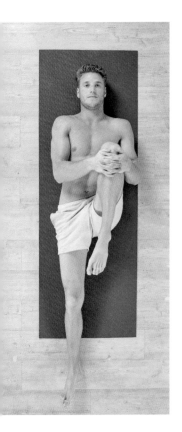

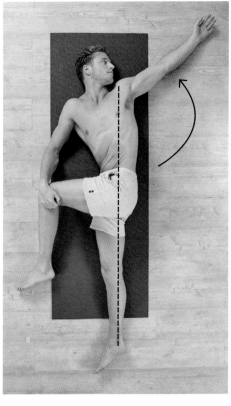

5. SIDE TWIST

In this exercise, unlike Exercise 4, you need to prioritise keeping the knee of your bent leg on the floor.

1-MINUTE MOVEMENT

Lie on your back on a mat with your right leg extended. Bring your left knee towards your chest and hold onto it. Turn your face to the right and use your right hand to draw your left knee across your body and to the right side. Firmly keep your knee on the floor. Extend your left arm out and to the side of your body, finding a point where the underneath of your shoulder is in contact with the floor. Turn to face your extended hand. **Slowly sweep your arm up and down for 30 seconds**. Prioritise keeping your shoulder in contact with the floor. Repeat on the other side.

1-MINUTE HOLD

For the hold, adopt the movement position, making sure that your shoulder is in full contact with the floor. **Take your straight arm out and to the side, finding a point where the underneath of your shoulder is in contact with the floor. Hold.** Pull your knee up towards your body for the most effective stretch.

HINT: The lower your arm is, the more likely you will be able to keep your shoulder in contact with the floor.

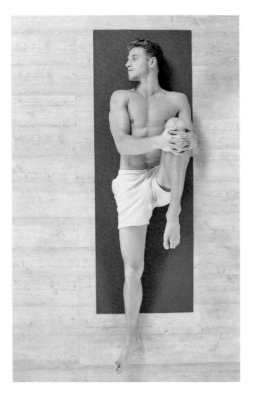

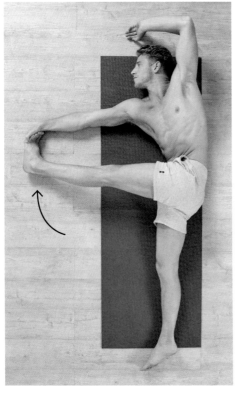

6. SIDE TWIST — STRAIGHT LEG

I came up with this stretch by accident when I was practising variations of the Side Twist. I suddenly felt the most evil of stretches on the outside of my leg as I locked it straight.

1-MINUTE MOVEMENT

Set up your regular side twist (opposite), beginning by crossing your left leg over your body to your right side. Press your knee to the floor, and stretch out your left arm to the side and up, turning your face to look at your outstretched hand. Now, take hold of your left toes with your right hand, keeping your leg bent. **Slowly straighten your left leg over 30 seconds, keeping hold of your foot**. Swap sides and repeat.

NOTE: You may find there is no way at this point you can get your leg straight. If so, just straighten as much as you can for now.

1-MINUTE HOLD

Starting in the Side Twist (as above), **straighten your leg and hold**. To increase the stretch, straighten your free arm out to the side opposite, and turn to look at your hand, aiming to get your shoulder in contact with the floor. Hold for 30 seconds, then swap sides.

9. HIP-OPENER ROCKS

The dreaded Hip Opener! Ever sat down in a chair? Ever run? Then this is the exercise for you. First, I must apologise for the amount of stretch you are about to feel: this one is certainly not for the faint-hearted. The aim of your exercise is to get your hips forwards — as far as possible without rotating them.

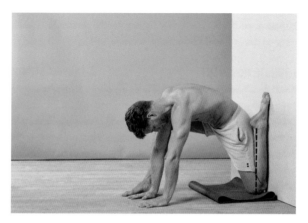

1-MINUTE MOVEMENT

Kneel on a mat with your back to a wall. Position your left knee and shin against the wall, toes pointing upwards. Place your right foot flat on the floor, leg bent at right angles for support, hands on your knee. **Move slowly between having your butt against the wall and pushing your front knee forwards for 30 seconds.** Swap and repeat.

1-MINUTE HOLD

Adopt the pressed-forwards position as in the movement, and hold for 30 seconds. Swap legs and repeat the hold on the other side.

REMEMBER: Press your hip as far forwards in the stretch as possible, being careful not to rotate your hips. Your hips should remain square and facing forwards. You'll know when you are far forwards enough because you'll be able to squeeze your butt.

ADVANCED EXERCISE: Sit up as tall as you can in the hip opener position with your butt against the wall. Move as far forwards as you can, one day aiming to get your hips to touch the floor.

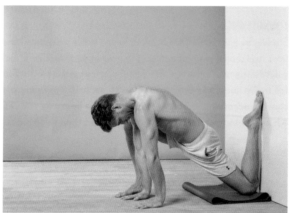

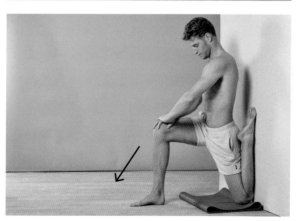

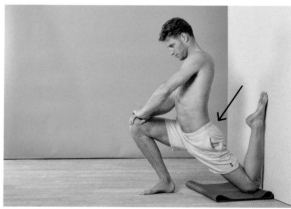

10. THE DEVASTATOR

For Exercise 10, I'm giving an advanced version of Hip-opener Rocks (see page 108). The back leg does the same in both, but the front leg changes to create either the Hip-opener or Devastator. Balance is important here so use two same-sized blocks or books for support. Eventually, you'll be able to do the Splits!

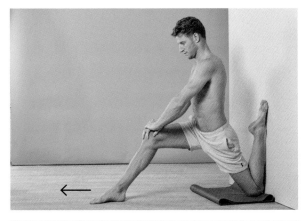

1-MINUTE MOVEMENT

Kneel on a mat with your back to a wall. Position your left knee and shin against the wall, toes pointing upwards. Place your right foot flat on the floor, leg bent at right angles for support, hands on your knee. Then, **slowly slide out your foot to straighten your leg.** Use blocks if you need to, otherwise **drop your hands to the floor as you stretch out your leg.** Reverse the movement, bending your leg again. Keep straightening and bending your leg, then swap and repeat.

NOTE: You must keep the knee of your back leg pinned against the wall. If you create a gap, you'll lose the effectiveness of the stretch.

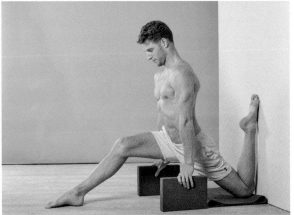

1-MINUTE HOLD

Adopt the starting position as for the movement. **Keeping your back knee pinned against the wall, straighten out your front leg and hold.** Swap and repeat.

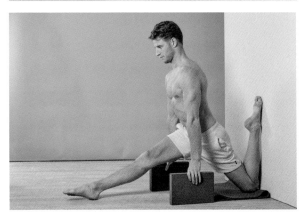

FOOD FOR THOUGHT

I've always found it odd in fitness and yoga classes when I've been asked to switch sides so that my body keeps in balance. We're not perfectly symmetrical, so why would you spend the same amount of time stretching the one side that you don't use as much as the other? A good way to resolve this is to start to become conscious of where you feel tight and work more on the tighter side. This way, your body will start to correct any imbalances and you can start to become in tune with what areas of your body are becoming restricted.

LIFE HACK

CHAIR STRETCH

Commuter Stretch (below) is probably my most frequent daily stretch. I can sometimes get an hour a day of this – in a meeting, on the train, sitting for lunch or dinner. There are so many times and places to get this stretch in what would otherwise be dead time. And the funny thing is, nobody has any idea you're stretching. In fact, you can almost look a bit slouchy when doing it. I've woken up in the morning feeling quite tight or sore if I've been driving or training the day before. After an hour on the train, switching legs at each stop, I feel really stretched out.

Remember to change legs. However, if you find you feel tighter on one side, perhaps you want to spend a little more time working that stretch. After all, most of us have dominant limbs, so it's to be expected that we'll be tighter on one side than the other. For more advice on how to do this, see www.roger.coach.

COMMUTER STRETCH

Sit in a chair. Take one foot and place it on your opposite knee (make sure it's the foot rather than the ankle), or higher up your thigh if you can. Use your hands to actively press down on the raised knee.

NOTE: The higher up your thigh, towards your waist, you place your foot, the more challenging the stretch will become.

FOOD FOR THOUGHT

We've discussed this before, but I'm going to keep saying it until it's drilled so far into your brain that it finally hits home. Your body is constantly looking for the easy way out. This is why when you get home you allow yourself to be lazy and slouch in front of the TV. When you step on that train, you robotically seek the seat. Being comfortable is easy. Easy doesn't get you anywhere.

I was listening to the conversation the other day between a married couple and one of them said to the other, "I can't bear the thought of becoming old. Will you come and visit me in my hospital bed?" *As though growing old and ending up in a hospital bed is normal!* This isn't normal. This is preventable. Yes, we all go through a natural ageing process, but some people decide to take action to slow down their physical decline. It doesn't have to be this way. Take action now.

What if every time your mind said, "I'm going to have a nice relaxed night," you replied, "You know what? Tonight I'm going to make a difference. I'm going to spend 30 minutes working on my body." I promise you, the feeling of satisfaction you get once you've completed this time will be amazing. You'll be so proud that you went against everything in your lazy mind and invested some time in yourself, and you'll feel a whole lot more energised than any night in front of the TV might give you.

What I mean by being uncomfortable is finding a sensation in your body that feels like a stretch. In classes, we're constantly reliant on the teacher coming up and showing us what we need to be doing. I'm inviting you at this point to explore your body for tight places, to not become reliant on somebody else to show you what to do. After all, nobody can feel what you feel.

As a coach, I can't guess what you feel; I can only advise on safe exercises that are easy to explain in the hope that this will guide you in the right direction. Only you will ever know what it "feels" like for you. There is no right or wrong in these stretches, apart from whether you feel good feeling or compensation (see page 29). Your body is *your* body. It is completely unique to you: where you're tight, other people aren't – and vice versa.

This book offers only a few examples of movements you can do to explore how you feel. There are millions of other exercises out there for you to try. Your body is your temple, whatever... just get the job done.

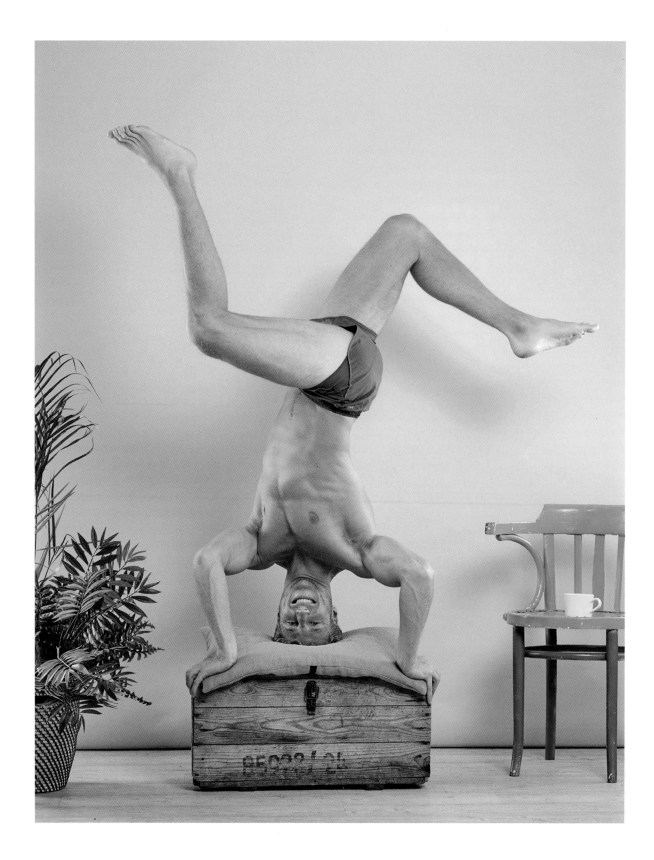

HEADSTAND

A good way to describe a gymnastic Headstand is an upside-down Front Support (see page 44) with three points of contact: one head and two hands. Of these three, the main points of contact are your hands. If you've already started working towards the Frog Stand (see page 70), you'll know I'm not a fan of jumping into position. The Headstand is not a balance exercise. It is an exercise of strength and skill. You'll begin to understand this when you start to lift into it using your core and utilising your hands.

If you follow the 10 exercises in this chapter in order, practising them religiously until you master each one, you'll learn how to support your bodyweight upside down. If you skip any of the progressions, please don't hold me responsible when you hurt your neck, back and wrists. Be methodical and rigorous – and a Headstand is yours for the taking.

BENEFITS

» Being upside can make you feel happy
» Full range of wrist mobility
» Looking great to your peers
» Shoulder and arm strength
» Great practice for the body line of the handstand
» Improved self confidence
» No more fear of falling
» Confidence at being on your head again
» An all-round fun exercise most people love
» Reveals the potential of your body

HOW TO MOVE

Choose 5 exercises from this book for your 10-minutes-a-day training. Identify the exercise in this section that you need to improve and repeat until you are able to progress to the next exercise. One exercise comprises both a 1-minute slow movement and a 1-minute static hold.

1. WRIST MOBILITY

When you do the Headstand, it's your hands that are doing most of the support. You will need to use your wrist strength as much as possible to make this work. It's a good idea to practise this exercise in front of a wall so that you can use the wall as a guide to the extent of the movement.

1-MINUTE MOVEMENT

Kneel on a mat, lean forwards and place your hands just in front of your knees with your fingertips facing you. **Sit back and place your butt on your heels.** Press your palms down into the floor to block them from leaving the ground. As you rock backwards, you should feel a stretch along your palms; if you don't, increase the distance between your knees and your hands. Rock forwards and backwards for 1 minute.

1-MINUTE HOLD

Start in an all-fours kneeling position, and turn your fingertips to face you. **Press your palms into the ground, lean backwards and hold.** Your arms should remain straight. Increase the distance between your hands and your knees if you can't feel the stretch in your palms.

VARIATION: If you find turning your fingertips towards you difficult at first, try them facing towards the wall.

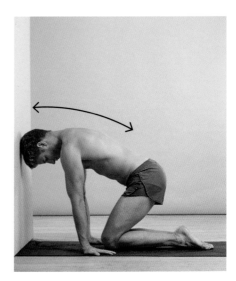

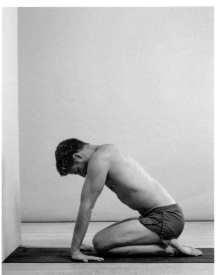

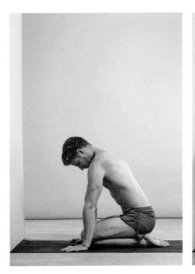

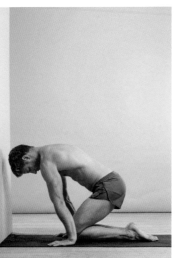

2. SETTING FOUNDATIONS

For Exercise 2, you're going to position yourself in front of a wall, with your head down, while your hands bear the weight. You'll need to press your legs straight while keeping your arms, head and elbows in the same place.

NOTE: Your head is up against the wall here – don't bring your head away from the wall at this stage, as this will cause you to roll on your neck.

1-MINUTE MOVEMENT

Position yourself on all fours on a mat in front of a wall. Put the top of your head on the floor against the wall, wrists beside your knees, fingers pointing forwards, arms forming right angles at the elbows. It can help to tiptoe your feet forwards before you straighten your legs so that your upper back can rest on the wall. However, if this causes more pressure on your head, take your feet back a bit. **Push into your palms, then raise your knees and move slowly between having your knees on the floor and straight legs.** Your forearms should remain perpendicular to the floor. Watch out for:

» Elbows falling to the side
» Hands too close to your head or too far back

1-MINUTE HOLD

Start with your head on the floor against the wall, and straighten your legs. **Hold your body in the straight-leg position.** If this is too much, bend your knees slightly. Remember:

» Head tight up against the wall
» Forearms perpendicular to the floor
» Elbows pulled into your body
» Hands firmly pressed into the floor
» Belly button sucked in
» Upper back against the wall

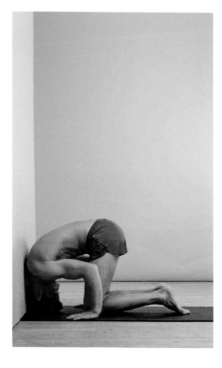
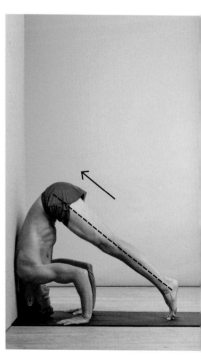

3. WALL SQUARE

For Exercise 3, you're going to bring your knees in on top of your elbows from the straight-leg position you mastered in Exercise 2. The starting position and checkpoints are the same as those in Exercise 2: head up against the wall, palms pressed firmly into the floor.

Some people experience pain in their wrists until their wrists and arms are strong enough to hold the position. Bringing your hands slightly closer to the wall should get rid of any pain.

IMPORTANT: As with all exercises, the goal is *not* to push through pain, but to learn about your body through the sensations you feel.

1-MINUTE MOVEMENT

Begin in the starting position for Exercise 2. Raise both knees so that your legs are straight (see page 115). **Bend one knee, bring it forwards and place it on the equivalent elbow. Repeat with the opposite knee.** Keep moving up and down for 1 minute.

REMEMBER: Press firmly through your palms to keep the pressure off your head and on your arms. Your arms should feel some fatigue after this exercise if you're doing it correctly.

1-MINUTE HOLD

Get into the top position for the movement. **Hold in the square position for 1 minute.**

REMEMBER: Make any adjustments that will help to alleviate pressure on your head and pain in your wrists.

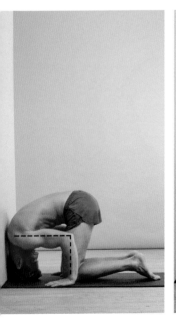
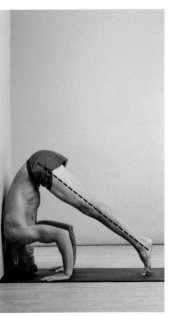
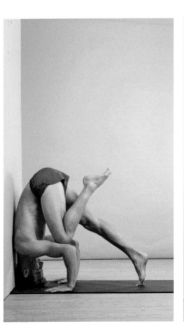
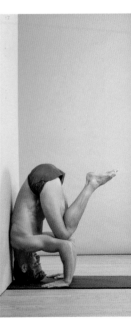

4. REMOVING THE WALL

If you've got to this exercise, I assume you've built a solid foundation for the Headstand by practising against a wall. Now it's time to remove the wall! Eventually, you will be able to hold your position for 1 minute.

1-MINUTE MOVEMENT

Use Exercise 3 (opposite) to get yourself into position but away from the wall: head on the floor, pressing through your palms, your weight supported by your arms. **Keep moving in and out of this position – knee up, toe down, knee up, toe down** – each time extending the amount of time you have both knees in position on your elbows.

1-MINUTE HOLD

Get yourself into position with both knees on your elbows. Hold yourself there for the full minute if you can (this will take time – don't worry if you can hold for only a few seconds to start with).

REMEMBER: The strength for this hold comes from the arms. Try not to just press your head into the ground.

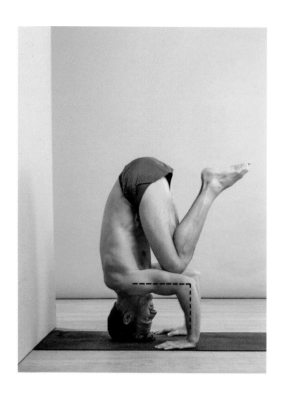

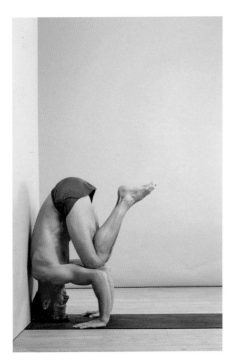

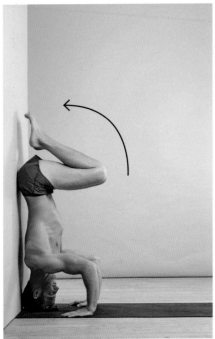

5. BUTT TO THE WALL

For Exercise 5, you're going to get your butt to touch the wall. You will do it by lifting using your stomach, which is easier said than done.

First, the stomach pulls the knees towards the armpits. Here, you really have to suck the stomach in using internal stomach (see page 59 in Hollow Body for an explanation of this). As you suck in the stomach, you press your palms into the floor and squeeze your elbows towards each other. You should experience your knees sliding towards your armpits. Another tip is to squeeze your heels towards your butt.

1-MINUTE MOVEMENT
Begin in the Exercise 3 (see page 116). Focus on the following points:
» Stomach sucked in
» Hands pressed into the floor
» Elbows squeezed into the sides
» Knees pulled towards the armpits
» Heels squeezed towards the butt

When you have linked all these points together, you will naturally rise up against the wall, moving through the transition position until your butt is up against the wall. **Move your butt back and away from the wall as slowly as you need to.**

TIP: You can see that the back is arched slightly in the second position. That's fine for now — we'll straighten up further down the line. Remember the aim is to get the butt to the wall.

1-MINUTE HOLD
If — and only if — you get your butt to touch the wall during the movement, hold that top position.

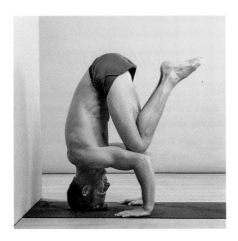

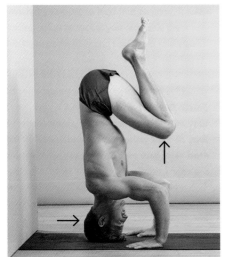

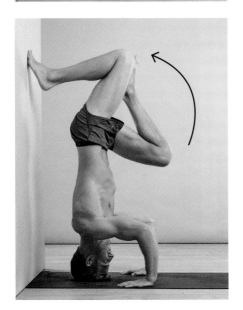

6. FOOT TO WALL

For Exercise 6, you've lost the wall again, so you'll need to become confident with Exercise 5 before you move on to this progression. This may take several months, but you'll get there.

1-MINUTE MOVEMENT

Position yourself in the square you created for Exercise 4 (see page 117), making sure you're in reach of the wall. Using the techniques from Exercise 5 (opposite), suck in your stomach, press your palms into the floor and squeeze your elbows to raise your knees. Once stable, lift one foot and carefully position it against the wall. It's common that your body will create a slight arch in your lower back. **Move between an arched- and flat-spine position.** To do this, you need to squeeze the knee that is off the wall into your stomach.

1-MINUTE HOLD

Move into the top position you achieved in the movement and hold. You can try 30 seconds on each leg, then move to the full 1 minute on each side. The most important thing here is the sensation you feel when you're in the right position.

9. STRAIGHT LEG, TUCKED KNEE

For Exercise 9, you're going to work up into a straight leg, so ensure that you're comfortable with the tuck versions before moving on to this. This is a controlled, conscious strength exercise, not a balance.

1-MINUTE MOVEMENT

Begin in the starting position for creating the square (Exercise 4, see page 117). From here, move into the tucked headstand (Exercise 8, see page 121). **Once you are in the tucked headstand, straighten one leg.** Once that leg is locked, point your toe and squeeze your butt on the straight leg side. Your bent leg will help you to keep the flat line in your spine as it is pulled in towards your stomach and you suck in. Return to your starting position and swap sides. Slowly straighten and bend for 1 minute.

NOTE: It's usual to adopt a slight arch in your lower back as you take your leg straight. Sucking in your stomach will help to correct this over time.

1-MINUTE HOLD

Bring yourself to the top position, one leg extended and locked, one leg tucked in. **Hold your body in the top position for 30 seconds.** Repeat with the other leg. You may find that you are constantly adjusting your position to achieve the correct line. I strongly suggest filming yourself or having a training partner to hand who can advise you on the position of your spine and the line from your head to your toe.

TIP: Feel free to upload a video of yourself to your YouTube channel, where I can give some quick advice. When I'm doing certain exercises and I'm unsure if I'm in the correct position, I will shout out things as I'm filming myself. For example: STOMACH IN, PELVIS FORWARDS, TUCKING IN KNEE, PULLING RIBS IN. Then, when I have a look back through the video, I can see which movements and directions are being the most effective in helping me to create a strong line.

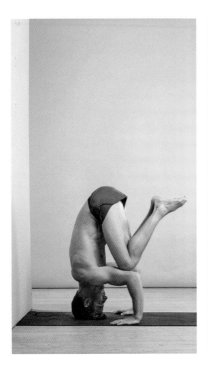
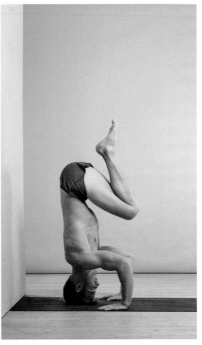
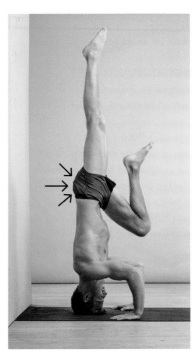

10. CORRECTING ERRORS

For Exercise 10, I'm giving you the two biggest errors you will come across in the Headstand, and I want you to use these positions to correct yourself into your line. The two biggest problems are:

1. PIKING
You have a strong line in the spine, but not enough forwards movement in your hips, which keeps your butt tight. A lack of movement in the hip flexors is often the cause – itself usually the result of too much sitting down. (To fix: sit down less and follow the exercises in Hip Action, see pages 98–111!)

2. ARCHING
Your hips are forwards and your legs are locked, but your legs are too far back because of an arch in your lower back. A lack of internal stomach strength or bad habits from performing the Plank (rather than the Front Support line) are common causes. (To fix: learn the Hollow Body on pages 56–69.)

These errors are, in fact, compensations – of reduced movement capacity or weakness, or even just a lack of understanding of how your body moves best. The good news is that the solid line is right in the middle.

1-MINUTE MOVEMENT
Lift up to your full Headstand using the method for Exercise 9 (opposite), but this time straighten both legs. See what position you go into naturally – are you piking or arching? Once you know what you need to work on, **use the Hollow Body progressions** (see pages 64–65) to obtain the correct position. Then, come back to your Headstand and try to mimic the movements you used.

1-MINUTE HOLD
Using the steps in Exercise 9 and everything you've learned in this movement, **raise up into a Headstand and hold your body in the correct line.** You will need a camera or friend to help you get the right position. At first, when you're holding the line, you'll find you are constantly correcting your position. Focus on the sensations you feel and this will give you clues as to what might be going on.

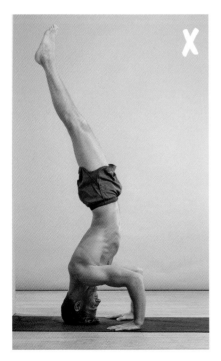
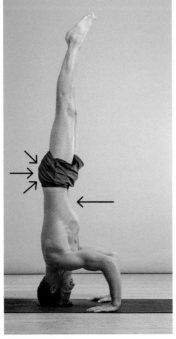
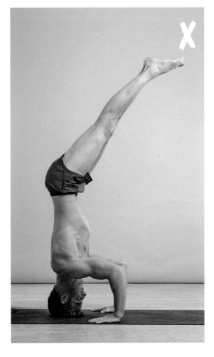

10 + TAKE OFF

If you've reached this page, I'm assuming you've mastered a couple of the bent-arm moves (Frog Stand and Headstand) so I thought I'd give you a little snippet of how to master the move on front cover.

I highly recommend mastering at least the Frog Stand (see page 71) before trying to lift off! I used a suitcase throughout this sequence to add stable height from the floor, but I suggest playing around with different items around the house to get used to what's going on in the move. Blocks, books, you now how we roll by now...

STEP 1. Start in a tiptoe squat position with straight arms (see Exercise 8, page 79).

STEP 2. Lean forwards, bending your elbows and squeezing them towards each other so that they sit directly underneath your hips.

STEP 3. Gently tip your bodyweight forwards until your head lands fully on the floor and you can rest on your forehead. Your elbows are still pulled into your body and are at right angles to the floor. Your toes are still on the floor and your knees are hovering just off of the floor.

STEP 4. Roll onto the top of your head slightly leaning your forearms forward as you do so. As in the Headstand (see page 112) remember you're always pressing through the surface you're working on with your hands and not your head. Your feet are now hovering off the floor as a result of leaning forwards.

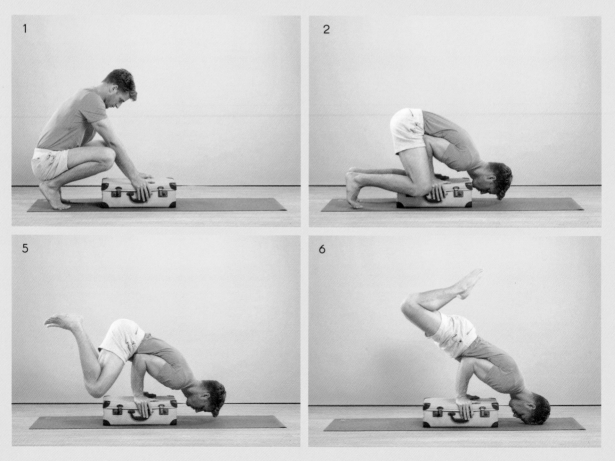

STEP 5. From here, unroll your head away from the floor and shift your forearms back so that your elbows are at right angles to the floor again, but keeping your knees and feet off of the ground. Now there should only be two points of contact – your hands should be pressing down into the surface and your elbows should be supporting your hips. This is essentially the what we call the "Hip Stand".

STEP 6. Lower your head back down to the floor leaning forwards on top of your elbows and rolling back slightly onto the top of your head. Once you have the third point of contact (the head) point your toes and raise your knees as high as you can from the ground. It will feel as if you're trying to get your toes to touch the back of your head. Your hips are now open.

STEP 7. Keeping your head-, hand- and elbow-position strong, slowly straighten your legs as wide as you can and squeeze your butt.

STEP 8. Only when you are squeezing your butt, roll back from the top of the head to the forehead to take your bodyweight back to your hands. As you do this, the legs will lower slightly and the head will float off the floor.

FOCUS ON:
» Pressing through the hands
» Leaning forwards
» Keeping elbows at right angles to the floor
» Keeping your butt tight
» Sucking your stomach
» Locking legs
» Keeping toes pointed

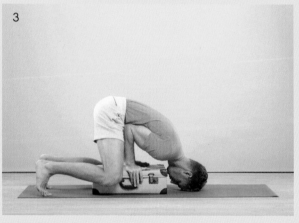

3

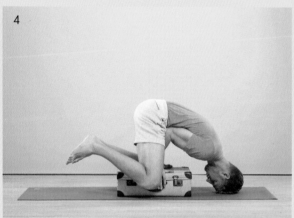

4

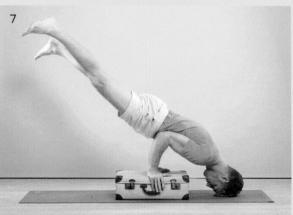

7

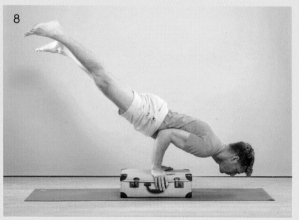

8

LIFE HACK

WRIST MOVEMENT

Q: How strong can your wrists become?

A: As strong as you allow them to become.

Your wrists, like the rest of your body, contain joints and muscles. You need to maintain them, especially if you want to do any exercises that put pressure on your hands, including Frog Stand, Front Support, Headstand, L-Sits and Stair Bridge.

In all these exercises, the only parts of your body in contact with the floor and taking the strain are your wrists. Ignore them and you'll end up with a very sore head and neck. I strongly recommend that you look after your wrists and make sure you're stretching them each and every way regularly. In return, they'll look after you. For more advice on how to do this, see www.roger.coach.

WRIST-BENDING

Become familiar with the mobility of your wrists. How much time do you spend with your hands in the same position? All floor fitness exercises tend to use one particular hand position. However, your hands can be bendy in lots of ways. If you're not completely comfortable with Exercise 1 of this series (see page 114), spend some time working on that before you try anything else.

FOOD FOR THOUGHT

» Suck in your stomach
» Point your toes
» Lock your legs
» Press into the floor
» Squeeze in your elbows
» Hold down your rib cage
» Squeeze your butt

...and all this while being upside down. This is where consciousness comes in – being aware of what your body is doing at any given time. "My back arches..," so suck in your stomach. "My head hurts...," so use your arms more and squeeze in your elbows. "My wrists hurt...," so, take your hands slightly forwards. Have you been stretching and strengthening them?

Pains and sensations are not problems but massive clues as to what's going on at any given time in *your* body. They are the biggest and most helpful giveaways, but *only* if you can note them and take immediate action to change what it is you're doing. Pain doesn't just occur, it occurs for a reason. Not only are you the only person who feels the sensation, but you're the cause of it.

You and only you can change it by having some long-term tools in place that prevent pain from happening repeatedly. However, those tools work only if you stop seeing pain as a hindrance and start to view it as a valuable tool in itself. Then, you can start the process of asking appropriate questions.

» Why is it that I feel pain when I do that movement?
» What can I change to make it feel different?
» How much am I even aware of *how* I'm moving?

Successful practitioners don't become emotionally frustrated or give up when they come across a barrier in their training. They don't just keep repeating the same thing over and over that is causing the problem; they don't go, "I feel pain when I do that movement, therefore I won't/can't do it."

Be smart about the issue. Don't instantly go off looking for somebody to "fix" you. Be conscious of the issue at hand and look for some resolution by changing or taking a different approach to what it is you're doing.

THE SAME OLD THINKING EQUALS THE SAME OLD RESULTS.
CHOOSE LIFE, CHOOSE CONSCIOUSNESS.

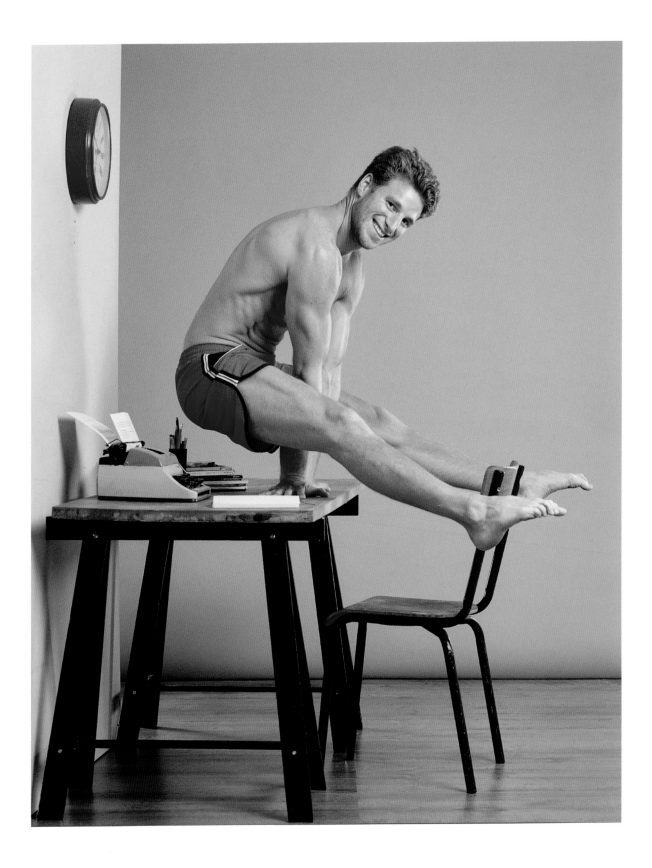

L-SITS

The L-Sits (straight leg and wide leg) – based on the ability to suspend yourself above the floor using your arms – are for me true tests of strength and flexibility, and require you to press through your shoulders to the floor and LIFT OFF! Don't worry. You're going to start by pushing against a higher surface than the floor. By the time you work your way to the floor, you'll have understood exactly what I mean by pressing through the shoulders.

Let's just get one thing straight: gymnasts do not have extra-long arms.

I remember when I first attempted an L-Sit. I was really puzzled as to how people were holding themselves from the floor, but as soon as I realised that I could do it, too, starting with a surface higher than the floor, it soon made sense. L-Sits are a long-term goal and will improve with time and practice.

First, you're going to start by using some tables, then you're going to move onto chairs and then onto blocks (or books). If you're working on a surface where you can hold yourself for only a few seconds, I advise you to start a bit higher until you're able to hold comfortably for at least 20 seconds. The key is to keep reducing the height of the surface you're working on until you reach the floor.

As long as you keep reminding yourself that good things take time, you'll be fine. So, let's get started.

BENEFITS
» Shoulder mobility and strength
» Leg flexibility and strength
» Hip flexibility and strength
» Back flexibility and strength
» Core strength
» Mobility in the shoulder blades
» Looking awesome to your friends

HOW TO MOVE
Choose 5 exercises from this book for your 10-minutes-a-day training. Identify the exercise in this section that you need to improve and repeat until you are able to progress to the next exercise. One exercise comprises both a 1-minute slow movement and a 1-minute static hold.

1. SHOULDER PRESSING

For Exercise 1, I've used two bar stools to push against. Random, perhaps, but I want to demonstrate the versatility of this exercise. Have a look around your house for some surfaces of equal heights, where you can support your weight with your arms.

1-MINUTE MOVEMENT

Find two surfaces that will support your weight and suspend yourself between them. **Push down through your palms, elbow pits forward, arms locked, and raise your feet from the floor.** You'll find it easier to leave your legs bent, but if you want something more advanced, stretch your legs out in front of you. You're aiming to move between elevation, where your shoulders move up towards your ears, and depression, where your shoulders move away from your ears.

1-MINUTE HOLD

Now try to hold the move with your shoulders depressed (away from your ears). **Push down into your palms and keep your legs raised together in front of you.** Support your body using your arms. Your goal is to stay like this for 1 minute. If you can't hold for more than 20 seconds, you will need a higher surface. As you get better over time you'll be able to use lower surfaces and then the floor.

ELEVATION (SHOULDERS TO EARS)

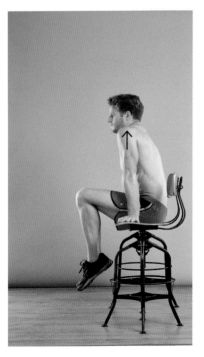

DEPRESSION (SHOULDERS AWAY FROM EARS)

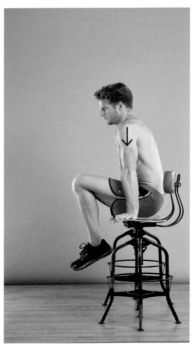

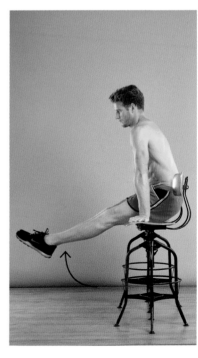

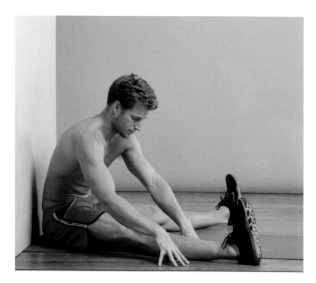

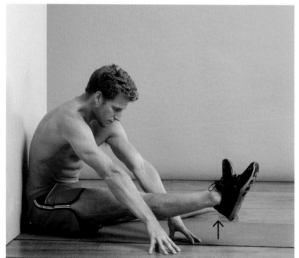

2. WIDE STRAIGHT-LEG LIFTS

For Exercise 2, you're going to experience what it feels like to pick up your straight leg. Since most exercises in the fitness world are bent-leg exercises, it can be a shock how hard this is. Press down through your fingertips into the floor on either side of your leg to help you.

1-MINUTE MOVEMENT

Sit on the floor in a wide-leg position. Place your hands either side of one leg. **Press your fingertips into the ground and lift that leg as high as possible, then slowly lower it back to the ground.** Repeat for the other leg, spending 30 seconds on each side.

1-MINUTE HOLD

Sit on the floor in a wide-leg position. **Press your fingertips into the floor either side of one leg and lift that leg as high as you can from the floor.** Hold, then repeat the hold on the other leg.

TIP: The closer your hands are to your feet, the more challenging the exercise will be.

PROGRESSION: Place your palms on the floor either side of your leg, rather than your fingertips, see photos below.

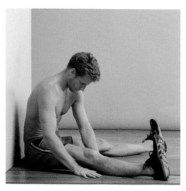
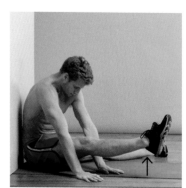

PROGRESSION: PALMS ON FLOOR

3. REVERSE PLANK

For Exercise 3, you're going to look at the Reverse Plank to see how your shoulders work when they are supporting you as you face upwards. The shoulders are the main element of support here.

You will have to press into the floor to get your shoulders away from your neck – the motion is back and down. Keep your shoulders directly above your hands, as you would for a forward-facing Front Support.

1-MINUTE MOVEMENT

Sit with your hands, feet and butt on a mat, knees bent. Press your hips forwards to raise your butt, squeezing your buttocks together at the top. Press your palms through the floor so that your butt presses up and squeezes to create the Reverse Plank line, but with your knees bent. **Roll down your shoulders, suck in your belly button and press your feet into the ground as you get to the top of the position.** Lower and raise for the full minute.

1-MINUTE HOLD

Press up to the top position and hold. Focus on:

» Hands pressed through the floor
» Shoulders rolled down
» Belly button sucked in
» Butt squeezed
» Feet pressed into the ground

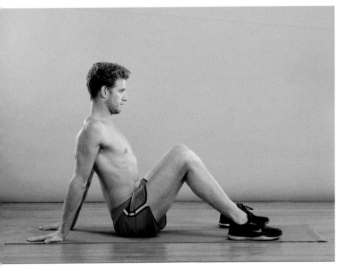
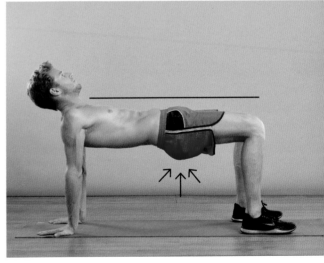

4. SHOULDER OPENER

Exercise 4 is a stretch with your arms behind you. It is designed to strengthen the muscles at the top of your back and stretch the front of your chest. Eventually, you want to work towards getting your hands together behind you, but at first, concentrate on opening the shoulders. If you experience any elbow pain, take the hands wider or turn the fingers outwards slightly.

1-MINUTE MOVEMENT

Sit on a mat with your legs stretched out comfortably in front of you, feet flexed. Put your hands behind you, about mat-width apart (narrower if you can), palms down, fingers pointing backwards. **Roll your shoulders forwards (internally; left photo) and then backwards (externally; right photo).** Repeat the rolls for 1 minute.

TIP: You can add more stretch to this exercise by bringing your hands closer together or by sliding your butt forwards.

1-MINUTE HOLD

Hold your shoulders in the externally rotated position. Keep holding for as long as you feel a stretchy sensation, which may be at the front of your body, around the chest area or around your upper back.

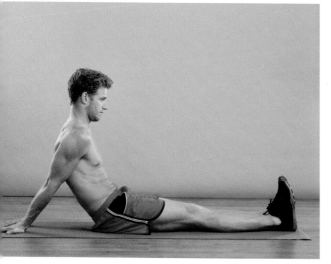
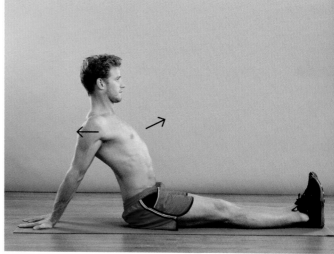

5. ADVANCED SHOULDER STRETCH

For Exercise 5, you're going to stretch your shoulders further.

During the exercise your rib cage is pulled in, like an advanced version of Front Support (see page 44), so you need to have mastered that.

1-MINUTE MOVEMENT

Sit on a mat with your knees bent, feet flat on the floor and hands behind you. Your fingers point backwards and your hands should be mat-width apart, or as narrow as you can get them. **Slide your hands away from you, keeping your arms straight and pull your knees off the ground towards your forehead. Bend your head to meet your knees in a straight line from the top of your neck to your wrists.**

1-MINUTE HOLD

Follow the steps in the movement, and once you have raised your knees off the ground, **press with your shoulders and use your stomach muscles to pull your knees in.** Don't worry if at first you can't get your knees to meet your head (good things take time).

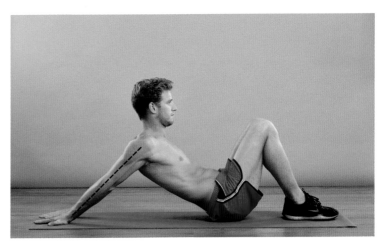

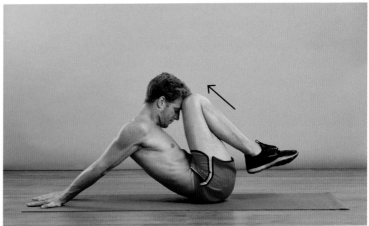

FOOD FOR THOUGHT

When you first start working with holds, it can feel extremely draining, and at times feel as though there is little or no progress. A good way to keep focused is this:"**Every second counts.**"

I really mean this. Every second of energy spent in the holds in this chapter counts towards the end goal. Just focus on one set at a time, 1 second at a time. Frustration and impatience are the enemy here. You have to know that every time you practise, you are improving even if you think you're not or you think you were better yesterday. Some days you're going to feel like you've slipped backwards, and you'll try to convince yourself your effort is not working. It *is* working. It *has* to work. This is the wonder of the body – our human ability to adapt.

It's just not a directly uphill journey. But that's like every journey and every challenge you'll come across – building a business, a relationship, a friendship, a life. It has ups and downs, obstacles and slow bits, but there is *always* progress.

I cannot tell you how many times I have practised a hold when out and about. Each and every one of them was just as important as any other; each a rung up the ladder of success.

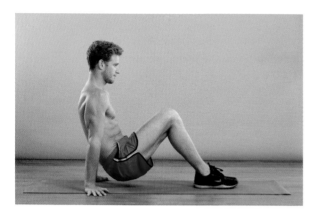

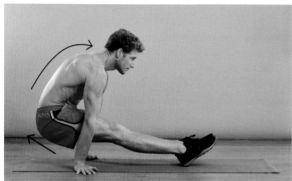

6. FOLDING PRESS

The Folding Press, for me, is one of the best exercises on your journey to obtaining the L-Sit. Think about this: gymnasts can press from this position into a Handstand. So, how do they get their legs through to the other side, let alone up into Handstand? Answer: they use their upper back and shoulders alongside a phenomenal level of flexibility. This is quite advanced so expect to spend a bit of time perfecting this movement.

1-MINUTE MOVEMENT

Use the starting position for Exercise 3 (see page 132), but this time your hands face outwards and your knees are bent. Keeping your thumbs forward and arms straight, **raise your butt just off the floor and straighten your legs**, sucking in your stomach, leaning your shoulders forwards and straightening your legs. If you can get your legs straight, start the next repetition with your feet closer towards your raised butt. If you can't, move your feet further away until you can.

Focus on:
» Pressing through the floor
» Pushing back your hips
» Leaning your shoulders forwards
» Sucking in your stomach
» Locking your legs

1-MINUTE HOLD

Put your body into the straight-leg position, aiming to get your butt as far behind your arms as possible. Hold. You're attempting to:
» Keep your arms locked
» Press your upper back round
» Hold your legs locked
» Suck in your stomach

7. TUCKED SHOULDER PRESS

For Exercise 7, you're going to look at how your upper back moves in the L-Sit.

During the exercise, your upper back is rounded, or you could say that your rib cage is pulled in. Both are happening during this exercise, which is essentially an advanced version of Front Support (see page 44).

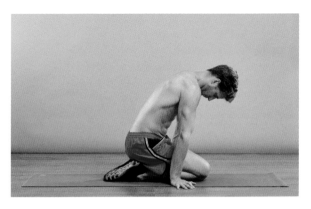

1-MINUTE MOVEMENT

Kneel on the mat with your knees just slightly in front of your hands. Round your upper back and press through your shoulders so that your shape looks like the photograph. **At the same time as pressing, pull your knees off the ground,** just enough so that you are on your tiptoes.

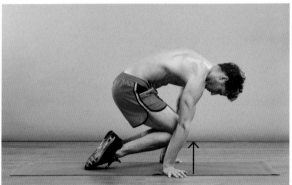

1-MINUTE HOLD

Once you have raised your knees off the ground, **press with your shoulders and use your stomach muscles to pull your knees into your stomach.** Try to concentrate on rounding your upper back to make your body taller. Your upper back should eventually stay rounded for the entire minute.

PROGRESSION: Eventually, you will feel strong enough to lift your feet from the ground in the hold for this movement. Don't attempt it until you can hold for a full minute with your feet on the ground.

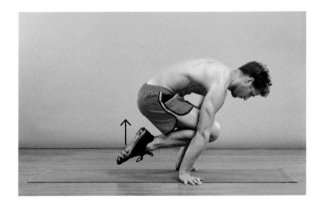

PROGRESSION: FEET OFF FLOOR

8. WALL FOLDING

A yoga teacher in a Yin class introduced me to this exercise as a relaxing way to stretch the back of my body. "Relaxing? This is so intense!" was my response. But my teacher was right: after a while, when the tight muscles start to ease out, it does become relaxing.

1-MINUTE MOVEMENT

Stand in front of a wall, feet slightly apart, legs locked. Stand far enough away to give yourself room to bend over fully. Fold your body from the waist until you reach a comfortable position that also gives a decent level of stretch. **Keeping your legs locked and straight, slowly slide your body up and down the pose, using your arms, moving in and out of the levels of intensity.**

1-MINUTE HOLD

Take up the starting position for the movement. **Take a breath, and fold over so that as much of your spine is touching the wall as possible. Lock your legs and hang there.** You may feel stretches anywhere from the heels of your feet up to around your neck. As long as it's a stretchy sensation, feel free to continue to hold.

NOTE: In these photographs I've demonstrated an advanced wall fold. You're working towards this, but move your feet closer and further away from the wall as appropriate. Most people starts much further out than they think they can achieve.

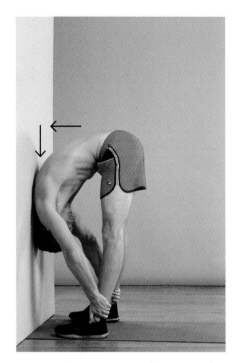

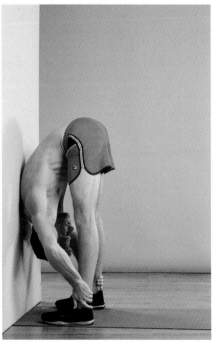

9. WALL PRESSES

For Exercise 9, you're going to use a wall to mimic the movement you will need to make when you press down into the floor to raise your legs. In the bottom photograph, you can see that I'm using my thumbs and fingertips to press into the wall at the same time as my feet come away from the wall.

1-MINUTE MOVEMENT
Position a mat against a wall. Lie back with your legs up the wall, then spread your feet wide. Raise your head and chest, reach your arms forwards and press your fingertips against the wall. **As you press into the wall, pull your legs and feet off the wall.** Release the press and relax them against the wall again. Repeat for 1 minute.

TIP: Try this with your legs at different widths: tightness in the groin will definitely restrict this movement. If you're struggling, the Hollow Body (see page 56) will help you raise higher from the floor, and the leg-flexibility progressions (see page 84) will help open up your groin.

1-MINUTE HOLD
Press into the wall with your fingertips and hold your legs and feet as close to your body as you can with your knees locked. You may want to bring the feet in closer together at the beginning; you are working towards getting your legs as wide as possible over time.

ADVANCED PROGRESSION: Try using your palms to push into the wall instead of your fingertips.

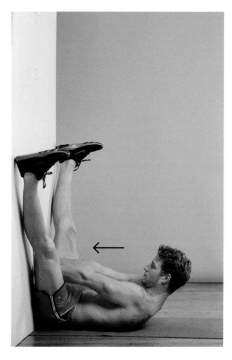

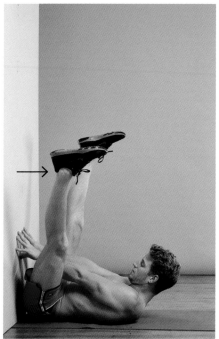

10. STRAIGHT LEG WORK

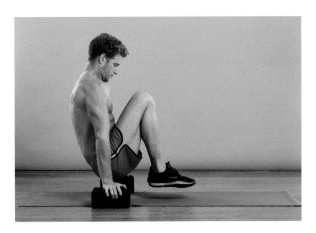

For Exercise 10, you're going to be working on the holds, but with straight legs. At the beginning, you will need to work on a higher surface than the floor to be able to get your legs straight. You'll need to practise getting straight legs both with your hands inside and outside your legs.

1-MINUTE MOVEMENT

Find two surfaces from which you can suspend yourself and that will take your bodyweight. You could use push-up bars, chairs or bar stools – it doesn't matter how far your feet are from the floor, as long as they don't touch it. Press your hands flat on the surface you have chosen. Press your shoulders down through your arms and hands and into the surfaces to suspend your body. **Move between bent knees and straight legs.**

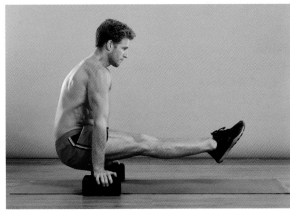

1-MINUTE HOLD

Adopt a straight-arm, straight-leg position, pressing with your shoulders, and hold. Hold for as long as possible during 1 minute. You should be able to hold at least 20 seconds in this position without your feet touching the floor. Once you can do this, you can repeat using a lower surface.

LIFE HACK: _____

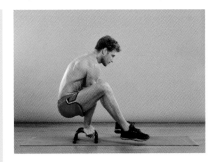

THE CHAIR AS YOUR SAVIOUR

So, how can we use dead time to practise the L-Sit? Remember that the objective you're working towards is being able to comfortably support your weight using your upper body and core. Chairs, unfortunately, are everywhere – they are responsible for more damage than any other piece of furniture. However, "why sitting down destroys you" can become "why chairs can save you".

Chairs, positioned either side of you, provide two brilliant supports, which act like parallel bars. You can practise a number of variations on them.

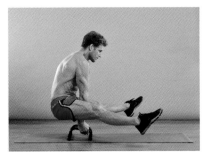

1-MINUTE HOLD

Find a chair that is safely fixed to the ground. Using your hands, press down on either side of the chair to either:

» Squeeze your knees up to your chest
» Keep your legs straight

Hold the position and repeat as many sets as you have the patience to complete. For more advice on how to do this, see www.roger.coach.

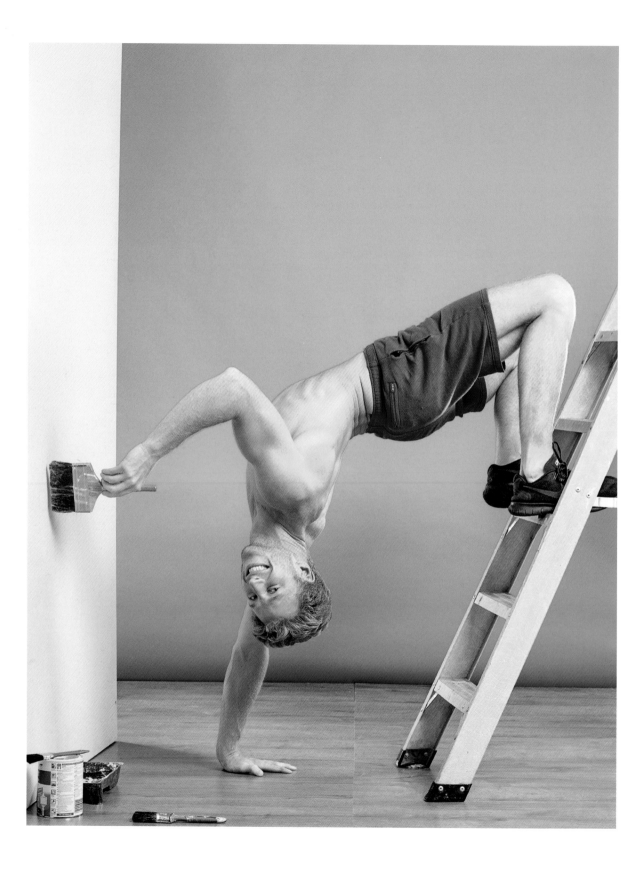

STAIR BRIDGE

9

The Stair Bridge is an overhead exercise designed to improve the flexibility of your shoulders and the range of movement of your spine. If you had a list of the most popular exercises you can perform, I bet they don't include one that teaches you to fully extend your spine.

Now, when I say fully extend your spine, I am speaking of the mid-spine, not the lower back. If you suffer from lower-back pain, it's important that you understand the connection. There are hundreds of causes of lower-back pain. One of them is that, through many years of sitting down, you've become very good at sitting in a flexed-spine position.

For example, the hunched-over, seated position results in a flexed spine that, in turn, has the potential to cause the middle of your back (known as the thoracic spine) to become tight and locked up. In effect, you lose access to it. We tend to use whatever is not locked up to achieve the movement. So, if your mid-back is immobile, what does your body do? It calls on the lower back to step in. Hence an epidemic of lower-back pain.

Largely there is nothing wrong with your lower back; it's just that you've lost movement from the mid-spine. The support exercises in this chapter will teach you how to start to incorporate some movement back into your mid-spine, because we have the support of our rib cage there, leading you literally through the steps towards Stair Bridge. If you feel pain in your lower back (or neck) during any one of the exercises in this chapter, you're feeling the result of a compensation. Bridging does not cause back pain. *How* you bridge can cause back pain!

These exercises suggest using chairs to add height to your movement. By lifting your feet from the floor, you will be able to achieve open shoulders in practising the Bridge. Eventually, you will be able to Bridge fully, from the floor, with no pain. (Stairs are ideal because they come down at even steps. I did it on a ladder, opposite, but don't do that; use something stable!)

BENEFITS
» Learn how to bend your back the pain-free way
» Overcome fear of being upside down
» Show off to your friends
» Improve shoulder flexibility
» Learn new skills and develop neural pathways
» Great for stress relief

HOW TO MOVE
Choose 5 exercises from this book for your 10-minutes-a-day training. Identify the exercise in this section that you need to improve and repeat until you are able to progress to the next exercise. One exercise comprises both a 1-minute slow movement and a 1-minute static hold.

1. BUTT SQUEEZE

The title of this exercise describes exactly what you're going to do. The purpose is to get you to start to utilise your butt muscles in order to support your back. With these muscles working to their full extent and purpose, you can eliminate tension from elsewhere in your body (mainly your lower back).

1-MINUTE MOVEMENT

Lie on your back on a mat, with your knees bent and your feet flat on the floor, shoulder-width apart. **Grab hold of your ankles, squeeze your butt muscles together, lift your chest and press your body upwards to raise your butt off the floor.** At the top position your butt muscles should feel tight and engaged. Lower a little if you feel any pain in your spine. You could feel stretches in:

» Your shoulders
» Your back
» The fronts or backs of your hips
» The fronts or backs of your legs

Once you've reached the top of your movement, lower again. Spend 1 minute raising and lowering in this way.

1-MINUTE HOLD

Using the starting position from the movement, **press, squeeze and lift your body into the top position, holding the squeeze in your butt at the top for 1 minute.**

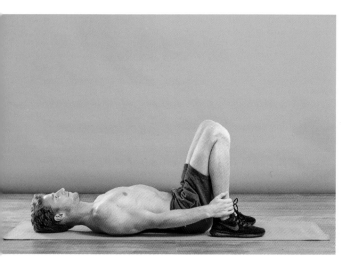

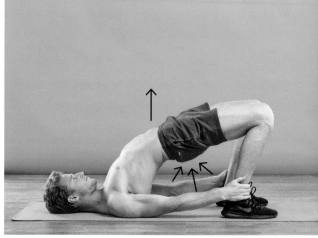

2. BUTT SQUEEZE, BOUND HANDS

In the last exercise, you grabbed your ankles and in this way you set up a good distance between your hands and feet. For this exercise, you'll need to bind your hands to help open your shoulders and add a new element to Exercise 1.

1-MINUTE MOVEMENT

Lie on your back on a mat, with your knees bent and your feet flat on the floor, shoulder-width apart. Press your feet into the floor and raise your butt a little. **Interlink the fingers of your hands underneath your butt to "bind" them. Squeeze your butt muscles together, lift your chest and move up to the top position.** Release the squeeze and lower to the floor. Raise and lower for 1 minute, keeping your hands bound beneath you.

IMPORTANT: If your shoulders feel very tight, regress to Exercise 1 and grab your ankles again. Move on to Exercise 2 only when you're ready, over time.

1-MINUTE HOLD

Press and squeeze your body into the top position with your hands bound beneath you. Hold at the top position and focus on working on the two opposing forces, pressing your bound hands into the floor and squeezing your butt upwards.

FOOD FOR THOUGHT

There are two opposing forces at play in this exercise: your bound hands press downwards into the floor, and your squeezed butt presses your hips upwards. If you feel back pain it is likely that your hips are tight. Try some of the Hip Action moves (see pages 98–111).

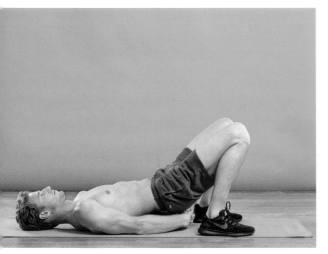
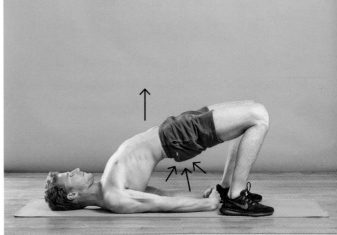

3. BUTT SQUEEZE, PLACED HANDS

For Exercise 3, you're going to progress exercises 1 and 2 – with your hands in place for the Bridge position. Your aim is to press your hands into the floor at the same time as squeezing your butt upwards. It's important here to establish a firm base of support with your hands because if the weight's not on your hands, it will end up on your neck.

TIP: You may find it easier to press your palms into the floor if you move your hands a little wider or further away from one another.

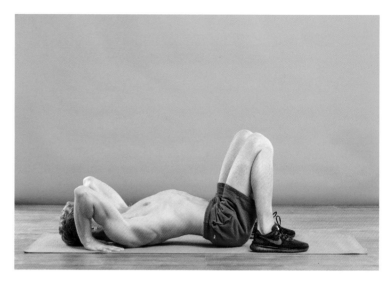

1-MINUTE MOVEMENT

Lie down on your back on a mat, knees bent and feet flat on the floor, shoulder-width apart. **Place your hands over your head and press your palms into the floor beside your ears, fingers pointing forwards. Press your hips upwards, lift your chest and squeeze your butt. When you reach the top of the movement, lower again.** Keep moving slowly between raised and lowered for the full minute.

1-MINUTE HOLD

Press your hips upwards, lift your chest and squeeze your butt. When you reach the top of the movement, hold. Pressing your feet into the floor helps to maintain the position.

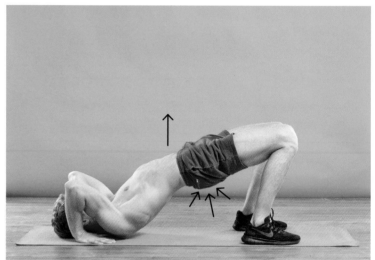

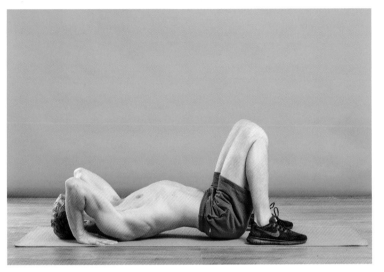

4. HEAD RAISE

For Exercise 4, you're going to take Exercise 3 just one stage further and lift your head off the floor. All the principles are the same as in the previous three exercises.

1-MINUTE MOVEMENT

Lie down on your back on a mat, knees bent and feet flat on the floor, shoulder-width apart. Place your hands over your head and press your palms into the floor beside your ears, fingers pointing forwards. **Press your hips upwards, lift your chest and squeeze your butt. When you reach the top of the movement with your head still on the floor, keep going. Keep pressing through and raise your head off the floor a little.** Continue moving slowly between raised and lowered for the full minute.

1-MINUTE HOLD

Press your hips upwards, lift your chest and squeeze your butt. When you reach the top of the movement, with your head raised slightly off the floor, hold for as long as you can, or for the full minute if possible. Pressing your feet into the floor helps to maintain the position.

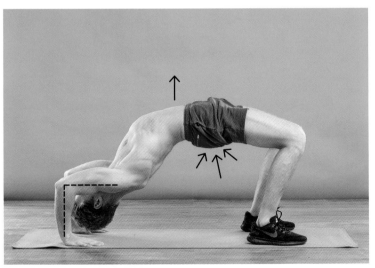

5. KNEELING TEST 1 – HEAD TO WALL

For Exercise 5, you're going to come away from your position on the floor and into a kneeling exercise, using a wall to test your shoulder and back mobility. It's essential in this exercise that you use the same motion as you've been using in the first four progressions. If you don't squeeze your butt, you're highly likely to incur back pain, and if you don't lift your chest, you'll end up just hurting your neck. Your neck travels only as a result of your chest moving.

The goal is not simply to touch the wall with your head, but to touch the wall with your head without causing pain. If you feel any pain in your lower back or neck, you must stop the exercise. This is not pain to push through. Creating more bend in your lower back avoids the expansion of your rib cage and only causes more problems further down the line. Back pain is a compensation.

1-MINUTE MOVEMENT

Kneel up, thighs wide, with your back to a wall, and your toes just touching the wall. **Bring your hands together in front of you for balance, then slowly and consciously bend backwards.** Keep bending until you can touch the top of your head to the wall (or stop if you feel any pain). **Slowly and consciously move forwards to the starting position.** Continue moving backwards and forwards for the full minute, as long as you don't feel any pain.

1-MINUTE HOLD

Starting in your kneeling position in front of a wall, lean back and touch your head to the wall. Hold this bend for 1 minute. You should feel muscular tension in your body, but no pain.

TIP: As you progress, you can start further away from the wall, increasing the backbend.

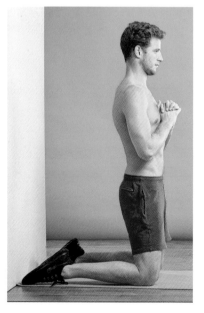
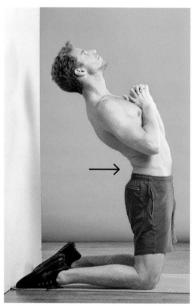
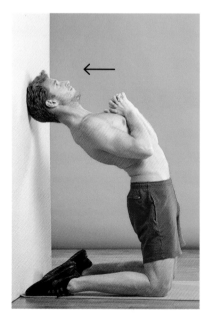

146

6. OVERHEAD REACH

Taking your arms straight and overhead adds a whole new dimension to the backbend. The tension increase will be quite dramatic from the kneeling version you tried in Exercise 5. I know I keep saying it, but I will repeat again: you should *not* be feeling any pain in your lower back here. If you do, it is likely that you lack shoulder or hip mobility, or both. Try the exercises on page 62–63 for improving your shoulder mobility.

1-MINUTE MOVEMENT

Stand with your back to a wall (close to the wall to begin with), feet hip-width apart, arms by your sides. **Stretch your arms overhead as high as possible. Then, lift your chest as high as you can, squeeze your butt to arch your back and aim to touch the wall behind you**, keeping your arms straight. When you've touched the wall, raise to standing again. Keep moving slowly back and forth, continuing for as long as no pain occurs.

1-MINUTE HOLD

Begin in the starting position for the movement, and follow the steps until you are **touching the wall behind you, arms straight. Hold.** Squeezing your butt and sucking in your stomach slightly will reduce the chances of you feeling tension in the lower back. Be careful not to overextend your neck.

TIP: You can make this exercise easier by stepping closer to the wall.

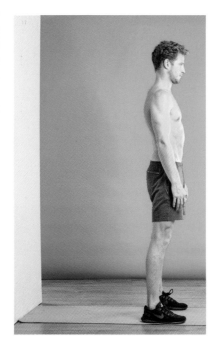
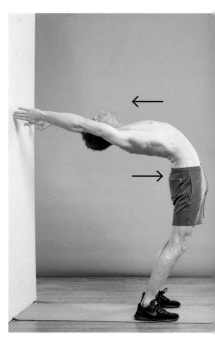

7. RAISED BUTT SQUEEZES

For Exercise 7, you're going to become familiar with how it's going to feel working on a chair or the stairs. Having your feet on a higher surface reduces the amount of shoulder flexibility you need to have in order to achieve the Stair Bridge. The exercise is more about becoming comfortable with that sensation and being conscious of the difference it makes to other sensations in your body.

Using a chair, which raises your feet, creates significantly less bend in the lower back than in the other backbend progressions so far. There's no need to purposely arch or straighten your back – just focus on squeezing and elevating your butt as high as you can.

Put your chair up against a wall to stop it moving away from you. Or you could use the stairs, if you prefer – just make sure you choose the stair at an appropriate height that doesn't cause any pain. The higher the stair you can manage, the easier it will be to transition into the later exercises. So, practise at different heights, but if one stair is all that's manageable for you right now, that's a great place to start. Take your time and progress slowly.

1-MINUTE MOVEMENT

Lie on your back with your heels up on the chair. Your butt should be close to the chair legs, bringing your thighs towards your chest. Hold onto the chair legs with your hands. **Squeeze your butt to press open your hips and raise your butt off the floor to its highest position, then lower.** Move slowly up and down, squeezing at the top.

1-MINUTE HOLD

Raise your butt as high as it will go. Hold at the top of the position for 1 minute.

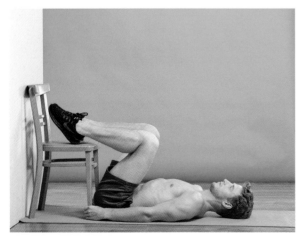
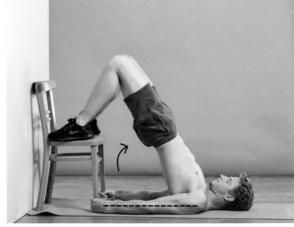

8. KNEELING TEST 2 – STRAIGHT ARMS OVERHEAD

For Exercise 8, you're going to create the same shape you made in Exercise 5, but this time with straight arms.

REMEMBER: Pain in your lower back is not something to push through. Creating more bend in your lower back prevents your rib cage from expanding and causes more problems further down the line. Back pain is a compensation.

1-MINUTE MOVEMENT

Kneel up with your back to a wall, knees hip-width apart, toes a short distance away from the wall. **Raise your arms above your head, reaching them as high as they can go. Once they are straight, squeeze your butt and lift your chest to move slowly and consciously backwards with the aim of touching the wall with your fingertips while keeping your arms straight.** Return to the starting position, then repeat the movement for the full minute.

TIP: As a progression, move further from the wall. One day, you can aim to move so far away that you keep moving backwards until your touch the floor. (I'm serious!)

1-MINUTE HOLD

Start in your kneeling position with your back to a wall, as in the movement. **Lean back so that your fingertips touch the wall with your arms straight. Hold this for the full minute.** You should be feeling muscular tension in the body. As you progress, move further away from the wall. Ensure the hips always push forwards.

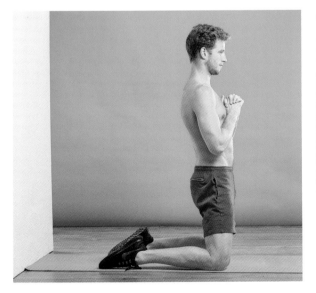

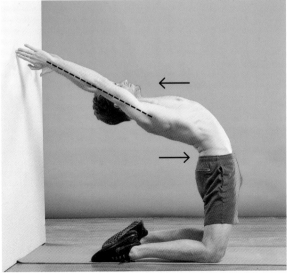

9. ARM STRAIGHTENING

For Exercise 9, you're going to place your hands overhead again. You'll recognise the movement from Exercise 4 (see page 145) although it may feel harder transitioning into this version, where the aim is to straighten your arms. Once you have your arms straight, there will be less pressure on your lower back from the action of lifting up.

1-MINUTE MOVEMENT

Lie on your back with your heels up on a chair or step. Your butt should be close to the chair legs, bringing your thighs towards your chest. **Place your hands over your head and press your palms into the floor beside your ears, fingers pointing forwards. Squeeze your butt to press open your hips and raise your butt off the floor to its highest position, press your hands into the ground until your arms are straight.** Move slowly up and down, squeezing at the top.

1-MINUTE HOLD

Raise up in the movement position as high as you can go and hold for 1 minute.

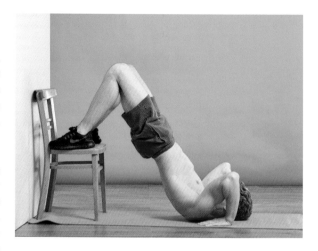

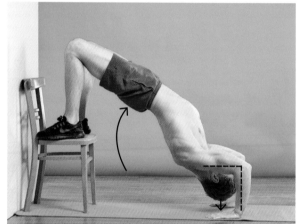

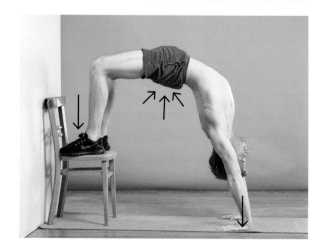

10. OPENING YOUR SHOULDERS

For Exercise 10, you're going to put all the progressions in this chapter together to create the Stair Bridge.

Like the other stair exercises, this is as much about being comfortable with different heights as it is about getting into the right position. The higher up your feet are, the better chance you have of being able to open your shoulders.

If your shoulders don't open, you will end up compensating in other areas (most probably the lower back or neck). Your lower back and neck have limited support, so it's important that you don't rely upon these parts of your body to hold you in position. You can't progress into a Bridge on the floor until you know for sure that you have full support in your upper back and shoulders.

1-MINUTE MOVEMENT

Begin in the hold position in Exercise 9 (opposite), with your feet at a height that is comfortable for you. **Press downwards through your palms to support you.** To get into the vertical line, three things have to all happen at once:

» Your feet need to press into the chair or step
» Your hands need to press into the floor
» Squeeze your butt

Once you have reached the top position, and your arms are straight, you will have opened your shoulders. **Bend and straighten your legs to bring your hips in line with your wrists.**

1-MINUTE HOLD

Press your body into the open shoulder position and hold. If you can't quite get the vertical line between your hips and wrists, you will need to take your feet higher.

TIP: Once you feel confident that you have your shoulders behind your wrists, you can start working your way onto a lower chair or step, until you can perform both the movement and hold from the floor without using any height at all.

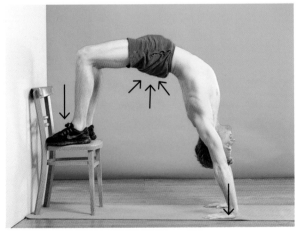
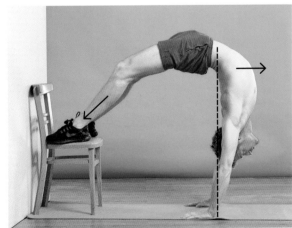

LIFE HACK

WATCHING TV

Have you heard of a yoga pose called the Sphinx? Picture a sphinx and you'll have a pretty good idea what it involves – lying on your front with your chest raised. Kids lie like this all the time. Good for them! It's a very smart way to open up the upper back. I'm going to give you a challenge: watch a TV programme all the way through lying in the Sphinx, then afterwards have a walk around the room to see how your spine feels. The position creates the direct opposite shape of how your spine is for most the day and it's a great way to slow down the ageing process in your spine flexibility. I wrote about 50 per cent of this book in this position, so I must thank you. Thank *you* for helping me to keep my spine open.

For more advice on how to do this, see www.roger.coach.

SPHINX HOLD

Find a comfortable place in front of your TV/laptop/book. Lie on your front, toes pointing behind you and raise yourself up onto your elbows. Look straight ahead. Try to keep your shoulders pressed backwards and downwards throughout the time you are lying there. Whatever else you're focusing on (your TV, your work, your reading and so on) will help to distract you from the sensations you feel in your spine and your rib cage will be open.

FOOD FOR THOUGHT

For gymnasts, a final Bridge requires the feet and hands on the floor. However, practising it if you have a lack of mobility in the shoulders, hips or spine can cause all kinds of problems, including neck pain, back pain and wrist pain.

This is the reason I will not begin teaching the straight-arm version of the Bridge with the feet on the floor. Raising your feet avoids unnecessary pain and strain on unsupported areas of your body, allowing you to progress safely without pain. Trying to get into the full version from the floor when you don't have shoulder mobility and don't understand how your tight shoulders hinder progress and damage your body. I know this because I did it that way myself for several years. This resulted in a very bendy and weakened lower back, which I spent lots of time reversing at a later date.

The Bridge is a wonderful exercise that will teach you a lot about your body. It deserves your full attention, and your patience when practising. Pain in any part of your body is a warning sign that you lack mobility elsewhere. Your body is extremely clever: it warns you when you have mobility issues, but you need to be conscious enough to receive those messages loud and clear.

Being conscious of *how* your body is moving is the key to progressing safely.

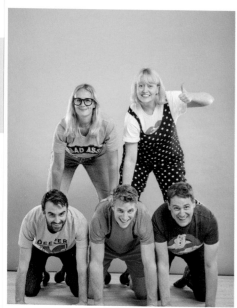
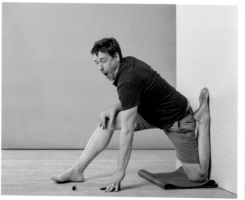
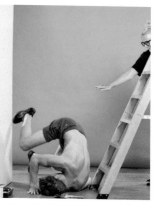
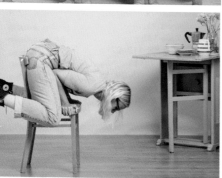
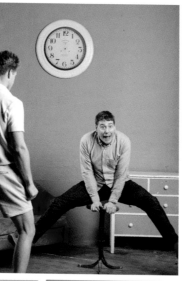
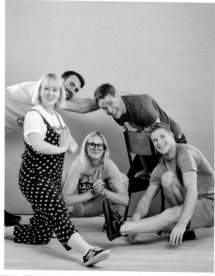
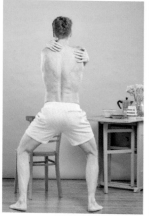
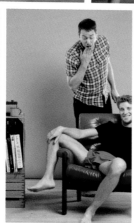
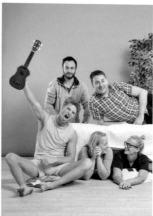
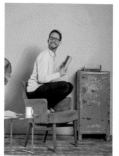
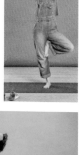

I had a lot of fun making this book and look at how well all the team could move by the end of it!

MY STORY

My story begins on a farm in England. Instead of watching TV and socialising, I spent my time exploring the farmland and taking care of business. Tasks included: building dens, clearing stinging nettles, removing misplaced logs, discovering old pathways, catching escaped chickens, climbing trees and picking apples. These tasks kind of became my job. Not because I was asked or told to do them, but because I really loved to do them. Hours would pass by as I beavered away.

Looking back, I feel quite lucky. I believe my childhood encouraged me to do things most kids would have never got the opportunity to do.

Then, when I was a teenager the family moved to East London. I want you to imagine this kid around 15 years old making up for a childhood without TV. I think in that year alone I watched every Hollywood movie out there. Jean-Claude Van Damme, Sylvester Stallone and Arnold Schwarzenegger were stars who became my heroes.

So I guess that was it... I had my mind set on becoming a bodybuilder.

I remember Day One of my attempt to get a body like Arnie. My local gym looked like it came straight out of a boxing movie: a converted garage space that had torn, black benches, rusting barbells and posters of ex-bodybuilding champions. The day I walked in there I met the owner – a proper Cockney guy called Dave. I described my health-and-fitness goals to him in great, lengthy detail just like an adolescent kid would: "I wanna get massive." He seemed to understand me. He pointed at the squat rack and said, "That there, son, is how to get big legs. That over there (pointing to the bench press) is how you get a big chest. And these dumbbells are for big arms, and that's about it. Now, off you go."

I became obsessed. I was at the gym five times a week with my piece of paper and a pen, ticking off exercises and writing down how much I'd lifted. My goal was plain and simple. You get the weight to where you need to get it to go and you've completed the rep. If you complete the rep, you move up in weight. As you go up in weight, you become stronger. As you become stronger, you get bigger... and you continue on this journey until you have the body of a movie star. Easy, huh?

It took more than a decade for me to realise that in fact, my body was far more complex than that.

In 2002, I was working on building sites for my father as an apprentice carpenter. I'm the sixth of eight kids and it was always my dad's dream to have one of us working alongside him. The apprenticeship was three years long. Close to the end of it, my sister had a party for her 30th birthday. There, I met Simon Harris, a photographer who took my life on a completely different course.

"Hey Roger, have you ever thought about modelling?" asked Simon. "No." (I mean, I really hadn't.) But, within a couple of weeks I was traipsing around London with a portfolio of freshly taken test shots, thoughts of a carpentry career left far behind. So what, you might say. Well, this switch from carpentry to fashion laid the foundations of the Frampton Method.

To be successful in the modelling industry (especially back then), you had to meet a certain size criteria. "What size do I need to be to be the most successful I can be?" I asked one of my agents. "32-inch waist, 38-inch jacket. And the better your body is, the more chance you have of picking up underwear/topless jobs." So, off I went back to the gym. But there was a problem. (I have to tell you this story because it's a bit of a shocker.)

I walked into my agency one day and the owner was standing at a table. I stood in the corner in my tight, white t-shirt, all pumped up from the gym, and she called me over.

"Who are you?" she enquired. "Erm, I'm Roger. Nice to meet you."
"Roger. Let me tell you a couple of things. First, never wear a white t-shirt if you're as pale as you are. Second, your face is a bit fat. Take off your top. Let me see your body."

So, I'm stood there in the middle of an agency with my top off, feeling really embarrassed.

"I like you, Roger, you've got great potential, but I'm giving you two weeks to sort yourself out. All this chest, arm and shoulder crap has got to go. If you want to make it in this industry, you need to get lean."

What a cow! Annoyingly, though, she was right. How was I ever going to fit the clothes if I continued to train the way I was? I was a 42-inch jacket and as stiff as a board. All I knew in the gym was how to get massive, not lean. So, from that day I quit weights for good. I'm proud to say that I haven't lifted a weight since – well, not for its intended purpose anyway.

Instead, I became obsessed with bodyweight training. Modelling wasn't as lucrative as I expected in the early years, so I got a part-time bar job and saved up for a diploma in personal training – and I absolutely loved it.

Everything I learned on the course made sense to me: you have days where you train your legs, then chest days, arm days, back days and, if you're really up to date with the fitness industry, you understand the importance of core and add a core-workout day to your regime.

I followed that methodology religiously for years. Until the day I walked into an adult gymnastics class and was ridiculed (again), this time by a six-year-old. She made me stop in my tracks. I'm talking about a light-bulb moment when something suddenly hit me and made me question everything I believed in.

Here was this young girl in a class filled with kids just like her, doing gymnastics right next to our adult class. She and all her classmates were able to move their bodies in ways that we adults couldn't. To them it was so basic – they seemed to look at us confused when we couldn't do the movements that they could do. Then, that six-year-old girl stepped forward and, at the request of our instructor, demonstrated to us what we were totally unable to do.

I sat there on the floor in this daze, exhausted from my shocking attempts at an exercise called a Bridge, and tried to cast my mind back to six-year-old Roger. I wonder: would six-year-old Roger be better at this than me? And if he were better, what had happened between then and now? Why had I become so bad at this exercise?

I started to research movements that are natural to humans as children, but that disappear from our movement repertoire as we grow older. One that kept coming up over and over was the squat. When I talk about a squat, the first thing people imagine is bobbing up and down frantically as fast as they can, but that's not what I mean. I'm referring to *sitting still* in a squat. If you want the correct terminology for this movement, try asking a four-year-old. They'll probably tell you that it's just "sitting" or "crouching", or maybe they'll just look at you confused. One thing I can assure you is that they won't tell you it's exercise!

If I could go back and jump into the skin of my four-year-old self, with the vocabulary and

understanding of my adult self, I'd look up at you and I'd say, "I'm just being human. I was born with the ability to sit like this. The squat is a natural human resting position."

Over the next few years, the discovery of the pure essence of what I call human movement would completely revolutionise the way I viewed exercise, the way I trained myself and the way I taught others to "get fit". I stopped exercising and, instead, I just tried to become four-year-old Roger again. I spent hours and hours testing the squat and other movements I'd discovered we were born able to do but had lost along the way. I used everyone I knew as human test cases — myself, clients, family, friends and colleagues. I was surprised to find that the majority of people I came across, even if they could do other movements, struggled to sit in the squat.

I now teach "human movement". Since that revolutionary gymnastics class, my only goal has been to "move like I once could" and to teach others to do the same. When it comes to this book, I'm teaching everything I've learned about movement and I assume that, because you've picked it up, you are human and you have some interest in maintaining your healthy human body until the end of time. Which is why it's so important to learn to move like a human again. So, this book is the next step on my mission to help you get back the movements you were born with.

You were born with the ability to relax in a squat, and if you lose that ability, there must be a cost that is restricting your movement; injuries, pain and potential joint replacements are inevitable in the longer term. However, if you put in some basic work on training your body to recapture some of your child-like flexibility, I promise that the chances of you needing a hip replacement or a stairlift will significantly reduce. I plan to have a healthy, moving body until the end of my days. This book is my invitation for you to join me on my journey.

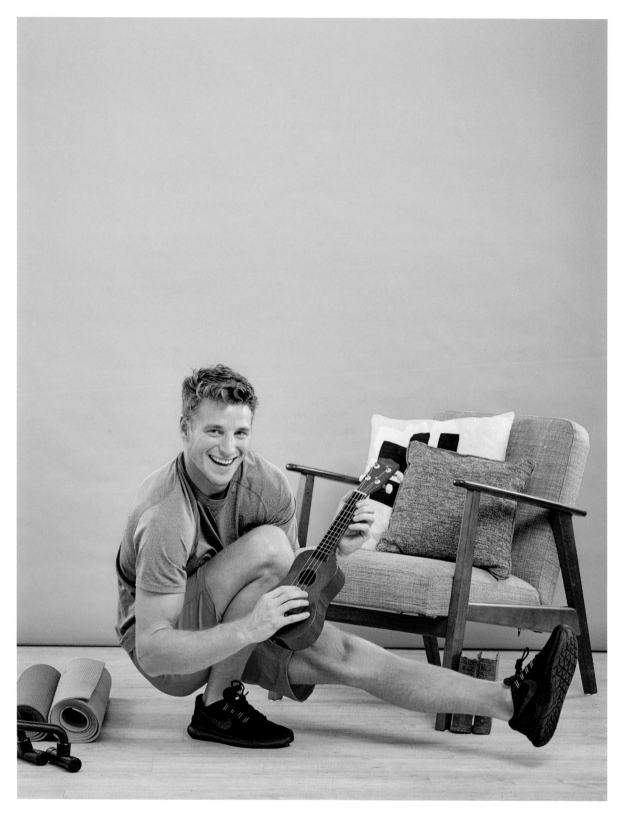

THANK YOU!

There are a few people I want to thank for making this book possible.

Firstly, me. That sounds a bit self-important doesn't it?! I don't believe you can take care of anyone unless you choose to take care of yourself and I'm advising you to take whatever you can from this book for the sole purpose of taking care of yourself before passing it on. We're conditioned to believe that the older we get the less we are able to move and this book proves that this doesn't have to be the case. A change in our focus on how we move will allow each of us to lead longer, healthier lives. So I thank me for making it a priority to take care of myself. Now it's your turn.

My parents. If my mum and dad didn't bring me into this world and work their arses off to make sure I way always fed and clothed then I wouldn't be here to tell my story and pass on my knowledge to the world. Thanks mum and dad.

My seven siblings (yes, seven!). Having a support network of best friends means I'm very lucky to always have someone there for me when life's not going as smoothly as I'd like it to. It's something that I am forever grateful for. Freddie, Gloria, David, Joel, Jane, Phoebe, Peter. Love you all till the end of time.

Campbell (no, not the soup…). Around ten years ago in a small flat in London a conversation occurred between me and my uncle Campbell. "I'm really not sure what to do with my life," I said. My uncle replied, "What do you love doing Roger?" "I mean obviously I love training and people are always asking me advice on working out but that's just a hobby. I don't know what to do as a career." "Roger, most people dream of doing the job they love for a living, now stop prancing around on catwalks and go and do what you love!" It was from that moment that I realised what doing a job I loved could mean. To love your job means you don't dread Mondays and you'd happily do it on a day we named Sunday. Why? For no other reason than because you love it! Thanks Campbell. I'm forever grateful for your words of wisdom.

Izzy. If you ever decide to write a book you need to know one thing. That although rewarding it's going to be one of the most challenging things you've ever done. My partner, Izzy, has always fully supported my crazy schedule even if that means working 7 days a week and waking up before 6am most days, before coming home and writing through the earlier hours of the morning. Izzy not only listens to me jabbering on for hours and hours about the same thing (movement obviously) but helped me test every image and every angle in this book for days in a studio before the official shoot. Thanks from the bottom of my heart Izzy for helping to make this possible. Love you always…

My clients. I have spent years in London parks and in people's homes teaching the fundamental bodyweight exercises I present in this book. It is only through those people trusting my thought process and allowing me to coach them that have allowed me to excel in my coaching. It's weird how around 90 per cent of people I train are called Alex. So if I thank Alex there's around 15 people ticked off the list. Thanks Alex.

Brian. The founder of London Real and also one of my best friends. On a chance meeting in a London park we made a deal. The deal was that I teach him how to muscle up and he'd make me work my arse off to write a TED talk. Well, if it wasn't for me getting up on the TED stage that day I wouldn't have written the theory that this book is based on. Thanks Brian for always pushing me outside of what's comfortable.

Dominic. I met Dominic when I was first training people at home. Dominic and I instantly got along and he was extremely supported of the method I teach. Dominic was able to give me advice that completely changed the way I viewed the world and even the language I used. Thanks Dominic for showing me that anything is possible. It really is.

Ben and the team at Pavilion. After seeing me on the TED stage Ben believed I needed to get my message out to the public in the form of a book and put me in contact with the dream team at Pavillion. As you can see there are a lot of things that have happened in my life to make it possible for you to be holding a piece of my philosophy in your hands. Thanks to Steph, Tom, Laura and the rest of the creative team that have made all this possible. We had some crazy times in those studios.

They say every coach needs a coach. I've had a few. Thank you to Sainaa at The London School of Hand Balancing and Aerobics, and Yoga teacher Caroline Pegna, who has taught me much over the years.

You. I believe in a world where all chairs are removed from schools, that all kids keep moving as they are born to move and that all schools as a curriculum teach children how their body moves best. In buying this book you're making this dream a reality and I am thankful for you believing in me. This is just the beginning… see you in the next book!